PRO(
IN PI

G000071313

THIRD EDITION

PROCEDURES IN PRACTICE

THIRD EDITION

Edited by
NIGEL A SCOTT
Department of Surgery, Hope Hospital, Salford

BMJ
Publishing
Group

First published in 1994 by
the BMJ Publishing Group
Tavistock Square, London WC1R 9JR
Reprinted August 1995

British Library Cataloguing in Publication Data

A catalogue record for this book is available
from the British Library

ISBN 07279 08235

Typeset, printed and bound in Great Britain by
Latimer Trend & Company Ltd, Plymouth

Contents

Contributors

J Au, Senior Registrar in Cardiothoracic Surgery, Wythenshawe Hospital, Manchester

PC Barnes, Consultant Physician, Hope Hospital, Salford

SE Beach, Directorate Pharmacist, Royal South Hampshire Hospital, Southampton

TH Brown, Senior Registrar in Surgery, Hope Hospital, Salford

S Burn, Registrar in Cardiothoracic Medicine, Hope Hospital, Salford

S Carne, General Practitioner, London

B Cramer, Consultant Radiologist, Department of Radiology, Janeway Child Health Centre, St John's, Newfoundland

JR Curtis, Consultant Nephrologist and Senior Lecturer, Charing Cross and Westminster Medical School, London

G De Lacey, Consultant Radiologist, Northwick Park Hospital, Harrow

PA Driscoll, Senior Lecturer and Honorary Consultant in Accident and Emergency Medicine, Hope Hospital, Salford

H Ellis, Professor, University Clinical Anatomist, Division of Anatomy and Cell Biology, University Medical and Dental School, Guy's and St Thomas's Hospital, London

E Forsythe, formerly Senior Clinical Medical Officer, Norwich HA, Wenhaston, Halesworth, Suffolk

AA Gehani, Senior Research Fellow in Cardiology, Hull Royal Infirmary, Hull

NJR George, Senior Lecturer in Urology, Withington Hospital, Manchester

JM Gumpel, Consultant Rheumatologist, Northwick Park Hospital, Harrow

A Higham, Clinical Lecturer in Medicine, University of Manchester, Hope Hospital, Salford

AV Hoffbrand, Professor of Haematology, Royal Free Hospital, London

T Hooper, Senior Lecturer in Cardiothoracic Surgery, Wythenshawe Hospital, Manchester

CONTRIBUTORS

S Hughes, Sister, Department of Surgery, Hope Hospital, Salford
PB Iles, Consultant Physician, Department of Respiratory Medicine, Dudley Road Hospital, Birmingham
PPB James, Honorary Senior Registrar in Medical Oncology, Royal Southampton Hospital, Southampton
DJ Jones, Consultant Surgeon, Department of General Surgery, Wythenshawe Hospital, Manchester
JC Kingswood, Consultant Physician, Trafford Department of Renal Medicine, Royal Sussex County Hospital, Brighton
S Kumar, Senior Registrar, Department of Respiratory Medicine, Dudley Road Hospital, Birmingham
IP Latto, Consultant Anaesthetist, University Hospital of Wales, Cardiff
J Luken, Nurse Specialist in IV Therapy, Royal South Hampshire Hospital, Southampton
ER Maher, Senior Lecturer, Department of Clinical Genetics, Addenbrooke's Hospital, Cambridge
AB Mehta, Consultant Haematologist, Royal Free Hospital, London
J Middleton, Nurse Specialist in IV Therapy, Royal South Hampshire Hospital, Southampton
C Noble-Jamieson, Consultant Paediatrician, West Suffolk Hospital, Bury St Edmunds, Suffolk
A Paton, Honorary Consultant Physician, Oxford Regional Alcoholism Unit, Chadlington, Oxon
JMS Pearce, Consultant Neurologist, Hull Royal Infirmary, Hull
C Record, Part time Consultant Radiologist, Stoke Mandeville Hospital, Aylesbury
M Rosen, Consultant Anaesthetist, University Hospital of Wales, Cardiff
NA Scott, Senior Lecturer and Honorary Consultant Surgeon, Department of Surgery, Hope Hospital, Salford
W Shang-Ng, Consultant Anaesthetist, University Hospital of Wales, Cardiff
P Sharpstone, Consultant Physician, Trafford Department of Renal Medicine, Royal Sussex County Hospital, Brighton
AN Thomas, Consultant Anaesthetist, Hope Hospital, Salford
JRF Walters, Professor of Gastroenterology, Hammersmith Hospital, London

A Watson. Clinical Lecturer in Medicine and Psychological Medicine, University of Manchester, Hope Hospital, Salford

A Whitelaw, Consultant Neonatologist, Hammersmith Hospital, London

L Wilkinson, Senior Registrar in Radiology, Northwick Park Hospital, Harrow

CJ Williams, Senior Lecturer, CRC Wessex Regional Medical Oncology Unit, Southampton General Hospital, Southampton

N Williams, Tutor in Surgery, University of Manchester, Hope Hospital, Salford

Introduction

Practical procedures are an integral part of all clinical medicine. The skills required can only be obtained by experience gained under the careful supervision of a senior colleague adept at the procedure. The look and feel of these procedures cannot be achieved by simply reading a book.

However, to carry out a practical procedure safely, with minimum discomfort and to most effect, a firm grasp of the overall requirements of each procedure is required. Thus you need to ask yourself before a procedure, what are the indications for the procedure, what equipment is required, what pitfalls exist – how can I tell if the procedure is successful?

This book gives an overall view of 25 practical procedures, many commonly performed in hospital and some in primary health care. Each is described in detail by clinicians who perform and supervise the procedure frequently. The aim of each account is to guide you in the safe and effective employment of the technique described.

The procedures have been grouped into three main categories, although there is clearly no firm dividing line between each category. The first nine procedures have been grouped together as those that might be used in the initial assessment and resuscitation of the acutely ill patient. The second category encompasses ten procedures that are directed at invasive medical diagnostic techniques and therapy. The final six accounts describe minor surgical procedures and more invasive clinical examinations. In addition, an appendix describing the practicalities of aseptic technique and setting up a procedure trolley is included.

This book is intended to be of help to all would be and actual junior medical staff in most clinical specialties. It is intended to help the medical student understand how to set up a drip, the SHO to grasp the basics of chest drain insertion and cardiac pacing and to allow the trainee GP to revise minor surgery and proctoscopy.

If studying the phenomena of disease without books is to sail an uncharted sea, while to study books without patients is not to go to sea at all, to practise medicine without a sound knowledge of practical procedures is to be up the creek without a paddle!

NIGEL SCOTT
January 1994

Part I
The acutely ill patient

1 Resuscitation in adults

PA DRISCOLL

This chapter describes how the procedures associated with the management of a cardiac arrest in an *adult* should be carried out. It is essential that you learn these techniques before being faced with the real situation.

How to do it: basic life support

Basic life support (BLS) consists of securing the patient's airway and maintaining adequate ventilation and circulation without the aid of any equipment. In practice, this is carried out on all those who suddenly become unresponsive following a respiratory or cardiac arrest.

The SAFE approach

> **S**hout for help
>
> **A**pproach with care
>
> **F**ree the patient from danger
>
> **E**valuate the patient's responsiveness

Your first priority on discovering a collapsed patient is to shout for help. This is followed by making sure the scene is safe. If the environment is dangerous then the victim must be freed from the area without putting your own life at risk. Only then should you assess the patient's responsiveness by gently shaking his or her shoulder and asking "Are you all right?".

> **When there is a risk of cervical spine instability, the head should be immobilised (Fig 1). If there is an assistant, ask him or her to stabilise the head from below as this gives better access to the patient's airway**

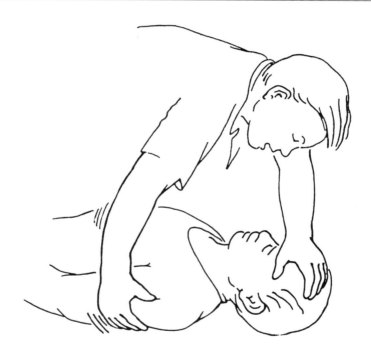

FIG 1 When there is a risk of cervical spine instability, the head must be immobilised while the patient is asked "Are you all right?"

If the patient gives a sensible reply with a normal voice, his or her airway is patent and the brain is being adequately perfused. Usually such subjects can maintain their own airway. However, a definitive assessment should be carried out, oxygen administered, and additional help summoned as required.

Assessing the ABCs

If there is an impaired response, shout for help and then rapidly assess the patient's **a**irway, **b**reathing, and **c**irculation.

> **A**irway
> **B**reathing
> **C**irculation

Airway

The most common cause of an obstructed airway is the sliding backwards of the tongue to occlude the pharynx. Other causes are vomit, trauma to the upper airway, or a foreign body occluding the larynx.

In most cases the tongue can be pulled forward, and a patent airway created, by using either a chin lift with head tilt manoeuvre or a jaw thrust technique. The cervical spine is not moved in the latter procedure and is therefore recommended in cases of suspected cervical instability.

In the chin lift manoeuvre, the index and middle fingers pull the mandible forward as the thumb assists and pushes down the lower lip and jaw (Fig 2). The jaw thrust technique is carried out by placing the index fingers behind the angles of the patient's jaw with the thumbs placed over the malar prominences. Downward pressure is exerted on the thumbs as the fingers lift the mandible forward. Again the thumb tips are used to open the lower lip and jaw (Fig 3).

If a foreign body is obstructing the airway then attempts should be made to remove it using a finger sweep, rigid sucker (Yankauer), or Magill's forceps, depending on the equipment available. Good illumination and care are necessary to ensure that the posterior wall of the pharynx is not damaged during this activity.

Breathing

The ventilation should then be assessed by placing your ear close to the patient's upper airway for 5 seconds. In this way you can look at the patient's chest for signs of movement, and listen and feel for expired breath. For obvious reasons this is known as the look, listen, and feel technique (Fig 4).

3

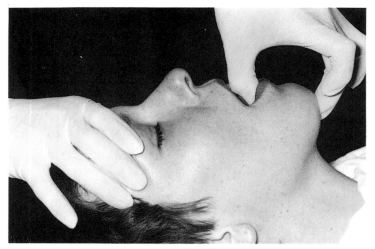

FIG 2   Chin lift

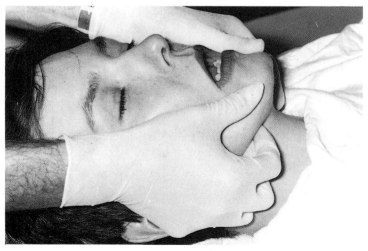

FIG 3   Jaw thrust

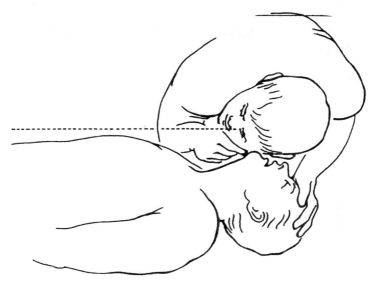

FIG 4   Look, listen, and feel

Circulation

Once the airway and breathing have been evaluated, the circulation is assessed by palpating the carotid pulse for 5 seconds.

Procedure

The subsequent management of the patient is dependent on the findings from the assessment of the airway, breathing, and circulation.

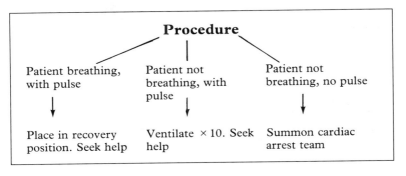

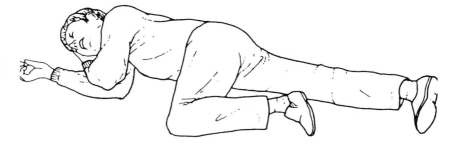

FIG 5   Recovery position

The patient is breathing and has a pulse

The patient should be placed in the recovery position and help sought immediately (Fig 5).

The patient is not breathing but has a pulse (that is, a respiratory arrest)

The patient must be ventilated 10 times by expired air resuscitation before help is sought. Mouth-to-mouth resuscitation is the most common technique and entails tilting the head slightly, pinching the nose, lifting the chin, and opening the mouth (Fig 6).

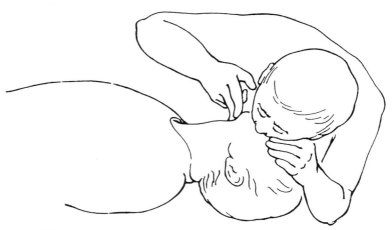

FIG 6   Mouth-to-mouth resuscitation while looking to make sure the subject's chest expands

You then take a deep breath, form a seal with your mouth around the patient's, and blow for 1–2 seconds. At the same time you should be looking to make sure the subject's chest expands. Between each breath the patient must be allowed to exhale passively for 2–4 seconds.

The patient is not breathing and has no pulse (that is, a cardiorespiratory arrest)

The only chance these patients have of surviving is early defibrillation. Therefore you must summon the cardiac arrest team, **even if this means leaving the patient.**

Once help has been summoned, full cardiopulmonary resuscitation should be started. In the case of a single rescuer, this consists of delivering two breaths followed by 15 external cardiac compressions. This ratio of 2:15 is continued **without interruption** until a defibrillator arrives or the patient spontaneously recovers. When there are two rescuers, a ratio of one breath to five compressions (1:5) is used.

The correct position for external cardiac massage is found by placing the heel of the hand two finger-breadths up from the xiphisternum. The other hand is then placed on top and the fingers interlocked.

Your aim is to produce sternal compression of 4–5 cm in the adult. To do this lock your elbows and position yourself vertically above the patient (Fig 7). Optimum compression can then be achieved simply by leaning forward and using your body weight. Reliance on the limited muscle power in your arms is liable to lead to inadequate chest compressions after a short period of time.

Precordial thump

- This can be of benefit in treating any ventricular fibrillation that has recently started
- Carry out if a patient sustains a cardiac arrest but it must not delay you from summoning help
- Carry out only once
- Hit the lower third of the sternum with the edge of your fist from a height of about 45 cm
- Start basic life support if there is no spontaneous restoration of respiration or cardiac output does not occur

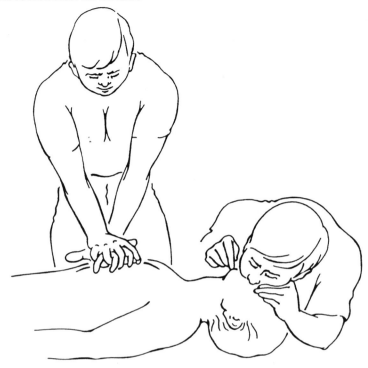

FIG 7   Position for external massage and mouth-to-mouth resuscitation

Chest compressions should be applied at a rate of 80/min. This can be controlled by counting aloud "one and two and three . . . ".

How to do it: airway management and ventilatory support

The most important aspect in the management of any patient is to ensure that the airway is clear and secure.

> **It is essential that you start with basic manoeuvres and assess the response**

Only if these manoeuvres fail, or prove inadequate, do you move on to more advanced techniques.

Airway adjuncts

If the basic airway management described previously fails, an airway adjunct will be necessary. The appropriate type of adjunct is dependent on the presence or absence of cough and gag reflexes.

A nasopharyngeal airway should be used if pharyngeal reflexes are still present. The size of this airway relates to its internal diameter in millimetres, with recommended sizes being 7 mm for a man and 6 mm for a woman. A well lubricated tube is inserted into a patent nostril and pushed backwards, parallel to the hard palate, with a slight rotatory action. A safety pin is then inserted through the end of the tube to prevent it being inhaled. Do not force the tube past any resistance as this can precipitate haemorrhage. The other nostril should be tried instead. This device is contraindicated if a fracture of the base of the skull is suspected.

> **The appropriate sized nasopharyngeal airway has the same diameter as the patient's little finger**

If the pharyngeal reflexes are absent, an oropharyngeal airway (Guedel type) should be inserted to help keep the tongue from sliding backwards. This type of airway is inserted upside down until the tip reaches the hard palate. It is then rotated through 180° and fully inserted until the flange lies in front of the lips (Fig 8).

> **The appropriate sized oropharyngeal airway has the same length as the distance from the corner of the jaw to the middle of the teeth**

Jaw thrust or chin lift can then be restarted and the adequacy of ventilation reassessed by the look, listen, and feel technique. Clear breath sounds on auscultation of the chest indicate that the chosen airway is appropriate and in the correct place, and that no complications have occurred.

Ventilatory support

Spontaneous ventilation

A close fitting mask should be placed over the patient's nose and

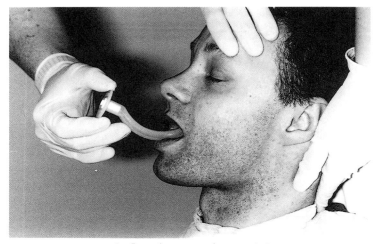

FIG 8   Inserting an oropharyngeal airway

mouth. To minimise re-breathing, and to compensate for any leaks, an oxygen flow rate of 15 l/min (litres per minute) should then be connected to the self inflating bag. Whenever possible, a reservoir bag should also be used as this will raise the inspired oxygen concentration to around 85%.

Artificial ventilation

If the patient is not breathing (apnoea) or has inadequate ventilation, then a bag–valve–face mask apparatus should be used to provide artificial ventilation (Fig 9). A one way valve prevents expired gas entering the self inflating bag. An oxygen supply of 15 l/min should be connected appropriately as this will increase the inspired oxygen concentration to about 50%. Whenever possible a reservoir bag should also be attached, as this ensures that the bag refills with a higher proportion of oxygen than room air. With a tight fitting mask this method allows the delivery of virtually 100% oxygen.

The facemask is held in place with the thumb and index finger, while the other three fingers perform a jaw thrust manoeuvre. The patient should be ventilated at 12–15 breaths/min (Fig 10). It is well recognised that a two-person technique, with one person holding the mask on the face with both hands and the other

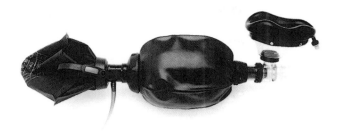

FIG 9   A mask, one-way valve, self inflating bag, reservoir bag, and oxygen supply

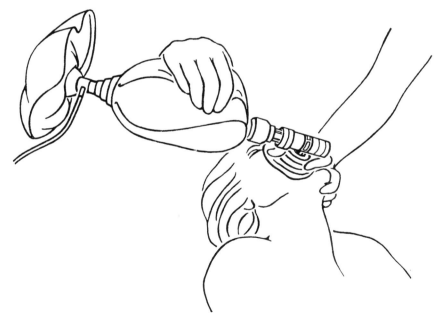

FIG 10   The facemask is held in place with the thumb and index finger, while the other three fingers perform a jaw thrust manoeuvre

11

squeezing the bag with both hands, is more efficient than a single person technique. If the situation and space allow you should use the two person technique.

Advanced airway control

In certain situations it may be inappropriate or prove impossible to maintain a patent airway by basic airway techniques (Box A). In these situations more advanced techniques should be used. The preferred method in the United Kingdom is orotracheal intubation.

Box A   Reasons for advanced airway techniques

- Basic control is inadequate or impossible to carry out
- Unconscious with loss of protective reflexes
- Poor airway with basic techniques – for example, severe facial trauma
- Specific need for ventilation – for example, head injury
- Compromise of normal respiratory mechanism – for example, chest injury
- Anticipation of airway obstruction – for example, inhalational injury

---

Equipment

Before attempting to intubate the patient, it is important that all the necessary equipment is laid out appropriately and checked (Box B). To prevent migration down the trachea and bronchi, loose teeth should be removed before intubation.

Box B Equipment required for endotracheal intubation

- Endotracheal tube:
    Male: 8–9 mm internal diameter, length 23 cm
    Female: 7–8 mm internal diameter, length 21 cm
    Check cuff has no leak and that the proximal end has a standard 15 mm connector

- Functional laryngoscope
- 10 ml syringe
- Magill's forceps
- Water soluble lubricant
- Functional Yankauer's sucker
- Bag–valve apparatus with oxygen and reservoir bag
- Catheter mount
- Gum elastic boogie
- Stylet
- Bandage for securing the tube

Procedure

Intubation must be preceded by a period of pre-oxygenation with a high flow of 100% oxygen using the basic techniques described above.

Whenever possible cricoid pressure should be used during the pre-oxygenation and intubation phases to minimise the chance of regurgitation and aspiration of stomach contents. It is carried out by an assistant using direct, midline pressure placed on the cricoid ring. This squeezes the oesophagus between the sixth cervical vertebra and the ring. The compression should not be stopped until the tube is in the trachea and the cuff inflated. However, the pressure must be released immediately if the patient *actively* vomits as there is risk of oesophageal rupture. In this situation the patient is tipped head down and the mouthed sucked out while cervical stabilisation is maintained. The patient can be turned on to his or her side only if a spinal injury has been excluded.

The optimal position for intubation is with the patient's neck flexed and the head extended at the atlanto-occipital joint (often likened to "sniffing the morning air").

13

The laryngoscope is lifted in the left hand and the patient's mouth opened with a scissor action of the right thumb and index finger. The blade is advanced down the right side of the tongue until the tip comes to lie in the vallecula. The tongue is displaced to the left. Force is then applied in the direction of the handle of the laryngoscope (Fig 11). There should be no wrist action as this can cause the upper teeth to be damaged by the proximal part of the blade.

This action brings the vocal folds (cords) and laryngeal inlet into view so that the endotracheal tube can then be inserted (Fig 12). Do not take your eyes off the target area until the tube is safely in place; a momentary lapse could result in the oesophagus being

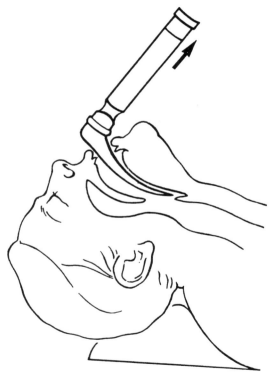

FIG 11   During laryngoscopy, force is applied in the direction of the handle

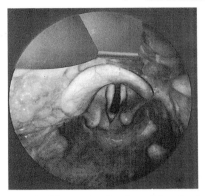

FIG 12   Direct visualisation of the glottis

intubated. If only the posterior aspects of the vocal folds are visible, a gum elastic bougie should initially be slipped through them. The endotracheal tube can then be guided over the bougie into the trachea and the bougie withdrawn.

The patient must not be deprived of oxygen for more than 30 seconds. Do not persist with the intubation attempt without intermittent oxygenation of the patient.

A tip is: take a deep breath when picking up the laryngoscope and, once you feel the need to breath again, so will the patient

---

Once in place the tube cuff can be inflated and the endotracheal tube connected to the bag–valve circuit so that the patient can be ventilated. The chest should be assessed for symmetry of air entry and the absence of gastric inflation. Auscultation should be carried out in the mid-axillary region to avoid being misled by sounds transmitted from the trachea. Air entry on the right side and not the left usually means the tube has been inserted too far. Check the length of the tube, deflate the balloon and withdraw it to the appropriate mark. If the correct tube has been used, withdraw it by 1–2 cm. Reinflate the balloon and reassess the air entry.

When there is doubt about the correct placement of the tube the cuff must be deflated and the tube withdrawn. The patient should then be pre-oxygenated again before another attempt is made.

Complications

Endotracheal intubation has several recognised complications (Box C). With proper training and preparation you can minimise their occurrence.

Box C   Complications following endotracheal intubation

- Trauma   Lips, teeth, tongue, jaw, pharynx, larynx, cervical spine
- Vomiting   Degree of unconsciousness misjudged
- Hypoxia   Prolonged attempt, intubation of the right main bronchus, intubation of oesophagus, failed intubation

---

A chest radiograph and arterial blood gas tensions should be performed as soon as possible after intubation: the radiograph allows identification of chest injuries and shows the position of the tracheal tube; the arterial blood gas tensions are used to check the adequacy of the ventilation. A large bore gastric tube should also be inserted to deflate and empty the stomach.

Occasionally endotracheal intubation is not possible because of oedema or trauma producing a complete airway obstruction. These patients require a needle cricothyroidotomy or surgical cricothyroidotomy.

How to do it: defibrillation

Ventricular fibrillation is the most common cause of cardiac arrests in adults and electrical defibrillation is its most effective treatment

---

As there are several kinds of defibrillator, you must familiarise yourself with the type you will have to use in the event of a cardiac arrest.

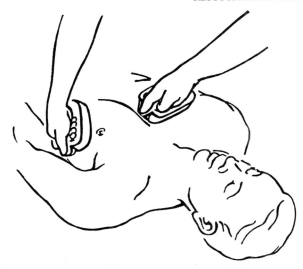

FIG 13   The common defibrillation position

Paddle placement

Usually one paddle is placed over the apex in the mid-axillary line and the other just to the right of the sternum, immediately below the clavicle (Fig 13). Rarely the anteroposterior placement is used. In this case the patient is rolled on to his or her side and one paddle is placed immediately below the tip of the left scapula. The other is positioned just to the left of the lower part of the sternum.

Safety

Sufficient energy is generated during defibrillation to cause cardiac arrest in people who are in physical contact with the patient. You must therefore ensure that nobody is touching the subject, trolley, or bed at the time the shock is delivered.

Procedure

The defibrillation sequence is as shown in the box on page 19.

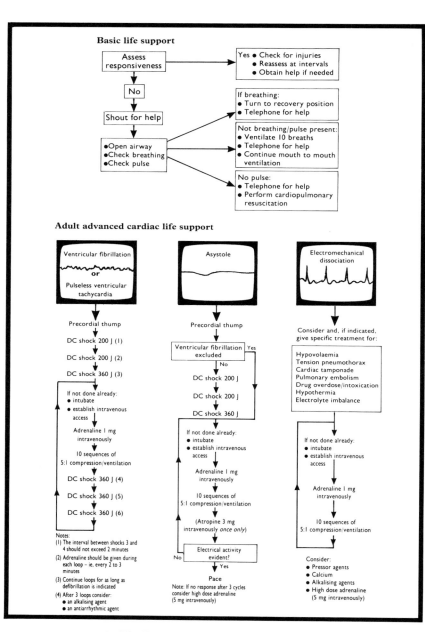

FIG 14   The European Resuscitation Council guidelines

Defibrillation sequence

- Connect patient to monitor
- Check patient and monitor – confirm ventricular fibrillation
- Apply gel pads to ensure good electrical contact
- Select the energy required (Fig 14)
- Press charge button
- Wait for the defibrillator to charge
- Lift paddles and keep thumbs away from the discharge buttons
- Place the electrodes on to the pads and apply firm pressure
- Shout "Stand back!"
- Check that all rescuers are clear
- Deliver the shock
- Check for pulse and check monitor

If ventricular fibrillation persists, repeat the above sequence until three shocks have been delivered. For safety reasons, the electrodes should be left on the chest when a rapid sequence of shocks is given.

Provided that the three shocks can be given within 30–45 seconds, then the sequence should not be interrupted for basic life support.

Putting it all together

The optimum way of managing a cardiac arrest situation is described in Figure 14. If there is more than one member of the resuscitation team, then central venous access and intubation can be carried out simultaneously.

Conclusion

This chapter has provided you with a simple guide to the resuscitation of an adult. However, it is important that you now practise, under supervision, the skills described. Your local resuscitation training officer will be of great help in this regard. In addition, all clinicians dealing with patients are strongly advised to attend an Advanced Cardiac Life Support course.

2 Peripheral venous access in adults

N WILLIAMS

Many patients have an intravenous cannula inserted as part of their management at some stage during their hospital stay, and this can be for a variety of reasons. Inserting such cannulas is part of the daily work of many junior hospital doctors. Obtaining venous access is a valuable skill which can be acquired only with practice. In some patients establishing venous access can prove to be very difficult and having a few "tricks of the trade" up your sleeve will not only prove invaluable but may prevent a blow to your ego!

Indications for venous access

Fluid replacement

This is perhaps the most common reason for "putting up a drip" and will be the main reason for the need to obtain venous access in a patient.

Drug administration

Intravenous administration of drugs provides the most rapid method of delivery into the systemic circulation of pharmacological agents. Many drugs – for example, antibiotics or chemotherapeutic agents – can only be given by the intravenous route.

Access

Some patients, for example after myocardial infarction, will have a cannula inserted electively for continuous venous access in case this is needed for the rapid administration of life saving drugs.

Feeding

Although most parenteral feeding is via a centrally placed catheter, short term administration of parenteral nutrition via a peripheral cannula is possible.

Indications
- Fluid replacement
- Drug administration
- Access
- Feeding

Types of devices

Venflon

This is the most common device used to obtain peripheral venous access. The indwelling part of the catheter is made of polytetrafluoroethylene (Teflon) to reduce the thrombogenicity and local irritant effect on the veins and so prolong its useful life.

Butterfly

These devices are usually for short term use only – for example, intravenous injections or taking blood.

Putting up a drip

To put up a drip the following (Fig 1a) are required:

- Cannula
- Infusion fluid already run through
- Alcohol-based skin swab
- Tourniquet
- Adhesive skin tape
- 5 ml saline for injection
- Local anaesthetic (for larger cannulas).

Running the drip through

> **Hint:** if you've never done this before observe one of the staff nurses to see how she or he does it!

- Remove all plastic coverings from the bag of fluid and the giving set.
- Close the valve for the giving set; then remove the protective cover from the connection points on the bag and the giving set.
- Connect the two devices using a screwing type action to ensure sound union of bag and giving set (Fig 1b).
- With the valve still closed, squeeze the bag to fill the chamber of the giving set by about one third. This will prevent annoying air bubbles entering the line when the fluid begins to run through.
- Open the valve slowly and allow the fluid to run through until it reaches the tip at the Luer lock connection.
- The giving set is now ready to be connected to the intravenous cannula.

> **Hint:** when about to give blood, it is useful to "prime" the giving set first with a 100 ml bag of normal (physiological) saline. This will prevent air bubbles in the line when you first start running the blood through

Problem	Air bubbles in the line
Solution	Vigorously tap the line and air bubbles will rise until they reach the chamber where they can be expelled or continue to run the fluid through slowly until all air bubbles are expelled

Choose a vein

> **Hint:** be choosy – give yourself the best chance

(a)

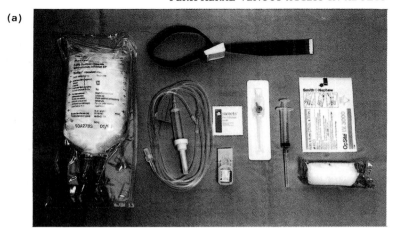

(b)

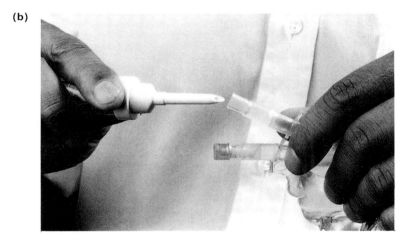

FIG 1   (a) Necessary items for "putting up a drip"; (b) the giving set being connected to the intravenous fluid

Assess both hands and forearms before deciding which vein to cannulate.

- Palpable veins are usually larger, have a thicker wall, and have more supporting connective tissue than veins that are visible.
- Cannulate veins at their confluence. This is particularly the case in old people who have less supporting connective tissue, and

therefore have frustratingly mobile veins which have a habit of shying away from your cannula. By cannulating at the confluence, the vein is more "anchored" and will not be as mobile.

● Try and avoid a cannula crossing a joint because this will almost certainly occlude on flexion.

In a few difficult cases the joint may have to be temporarily splinted to prevent flexion.

Problem   *No veins visible or palpable*

Action   1 Place both the patient's hands and arms in warm water

2 Come back and reassess after a short coffee break

Still no veins visible or palpable

Try a patch of glyceryl trinitrate over the most promising area and reassess later, or try using a sphygmomanometer cuff inflated to a low pressure, which allows arterial inflow, instead of a standard tourniquet

Still no veins visible or palpable

Call for help. Better to give the patient the best chance and also to save face

---

Choose the cannula

The size and colour of the cannula inserted will be governed by the intended use of the cannula and the size of the patient's vein. Cannulas are colour coded according to their external diameters. The diameter and length of the cannula have a direct influence on the flow rate that can be achieved (table). In general, green will be sufficient for the infusion of crystalloids, and grey and brown for rapid fluid infusion.

Insert the cannula

● The tourniquet is placed around the lower arm or upper forearm sufficiently tight to impede venous return but not enough to stop arterial inflow. Check that the radial pulse is still present.

● Ensure also that you have washed your hands and use an aseptic technique (see Appendix). Some units may insist that you use a sterile trolley and gloves; however, in many ward settings this is

24

Physical characteristics of intravenous cannulas

Colour	Gauge (French)	Length (mm)	External diameter (mm)	Maximum flow rate (ml/min)	Uses
Blue	22	25	0·8	31	Essentially paediatric use only
Pink	20	32	1·0	54	Paediatrics Difficult access Intravenous medication
Green	18	45	1·2	80	Most commonly used for fluids, drugs May be used for blood, though not ideal
Yellow	17	45	1·4	125	Ideal for elective blood transfusion
Grey	16	45	1·7	180	Allows rapid infusion rates, eg, obstetric and surgical patients
Brown	14	45	2·0	270	Major trauma, haemorrhage, gastrointestinal bleeding, etc

not always possible or necessary, although attention to asepsis should be observed.

- Having decided which vein is to be cannulated (Fig 2a), clean the skin with an alcohol based swab.

- There are many methods of holding the cannula before insertion and personal preference will prevail. However, the grip should be positive and allow control of the device during insertion.

- If a large bore cannula is being inserted then it is less painful for the patient if you anaesthetise the skin entry site. A small bleb (2–3 mm) of lignocaine is injected intradermally using a 25-gauge (orange hub) needle.

- Your non-dominant hand should firmly support the patient's hand (and if possible the thumb should stretch the patient's skin at the insertion site – Fig 2b) because this will prevent untimely withdrawal of the hand as soon as the needle is felt. This is an important manoeuvre and will result in more successful cannulations and a cleaner white coat!

- Once the needle has entered the vein, blood will "flash back" along the cannula. Gently insert both cannula and trocar a further 2–3 mm because this will ensure the cannula is fully intraluminal. The trocar is then partially withdrawn and the cannula advanced firmly along the vein.

- Remove or loosen the tourniquet before proceeding further. This will save on your laundry bill! Place a finger at the tip of the cannula to occlude the vein and prevent major backflow as the metal trocar is removed and the plastic cap fitted.

- The cannula should be flushed with normal (physiological) saline to confirm patency and satisfactory function, and prevent stagnant blood clotting in the cannula.

Secure the cannula

This is potentially one of the most important aspects of the whole procedure; a few minutes spent now will be valuable and can be the difference between a few hours uninterrupted sleep or being called to resite a cannula that has "fallen out".

- There are many proprietary adhesives or tapes and most are suitable. There are also some purpose designed dressings (Fig 3). Four strips of tape are usually adequate to secure the

(a)

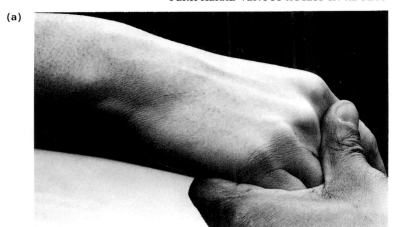

(b)

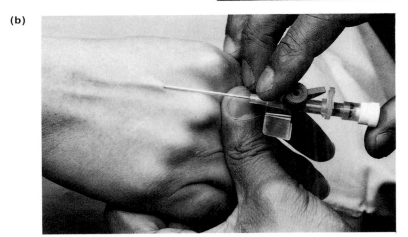

FIG 2   (a) Supporting the patient's hand before cannula insertion; (b) inserting the cannula

cannula. To prevent pulling on the cannula by the giving set, secure the plastic tubing with adhesive tape (Fig 4).

Sharps

- Careful handling and disposal of sharps are essential for the safety of all health service staff. The metal trocar from the

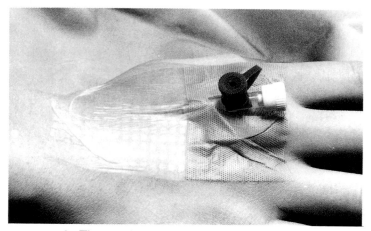

FIG 3 The cannula is secured by an adhesive dressing

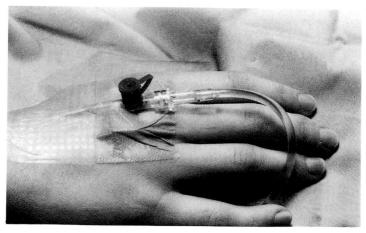

FIG 4 The giving set is connected to the cannula

Venflon device can be easily forgotten as attention is focused on securing and setting up the drip. Dispose of sharps carefully in a sharps bin. It is your responsibility.

Troubleshooting

No flashback
The likelihood is that you have not entered the vein. Do not remove the cannula. Withdraw it to within 1–2 mm of the skin puncture site and repeat attempt at vein puncture

Unable to advance cannula
Most commonly due to the presence of valves within the vein. Gently try altering the angle and direction when advancing the cannula. Alternatively, if the drip is connected and infusion commenced this may dilate the vein and allow further advancement of the cannula

Rapidly expanding swelling
This occurs if both vein walls have been penetrated (ie, totally traversed) or if a thin walled vein tears at the attempted cannulation site. It is almost impossible to salvage this situation. Remove tourniquet, remove cannula, and press firmly with a cotton wool ball at that site.

Known difficult patient } **CALL FOR**
No obvious access site } **HELP**
Struggling }

---

3 Putting up a drip and taking blood in young children

C NOBLE-JAMIESON
A WHITELAW

Putting up a drip

Intravenous infusions are often needed in young children and infants for rehydration, drug treatment, inability to tolerate feeding, and surgery. Modern plastic intravenous cannulas are small enough for use on limb or scalp veins in even the tiniest pre-term infants and have the advantage that they do not cut out of the vein even when there is some movement. The cheaper butterfly needle may still be needed for scalp vein infusions, although these should be avoided where possible as parents are often distressed at seeing hair shaved off.

Indications for intravenous infusion

- Rehydration
- Drug treatment
- Inability to tolerate feeding
- Surgery

Equipment

Assemble the materials for the drip in advance, in a room with a good light. The cannula used (22 or 24 gauge) should have short wings at the hub. You will need a strip of $\frac{1}{2}$ inch (12·7 mm) adhesive tape, a splint to secure the drip, and a 1 ml syringe filled with 0·9% saline to flush (Fig 1). A further syringe filled with

Please complete this card as it would help us to publish the texts you require.

Book title: ....

Where did you hear of this book?

Advert ☐ Leaflet ☐ Recommended ☐ Reviews ☐ Shelf ☐

How did you purchase this book?

Direct mail from publisher/bookseller ☐ Bookseller ☐

Did you purchase this book for

Individual use ☐ Library/department use ☐

What are your views on this book?

....

Do you consider the book represented value for money Yes/No

If not why ?

Please add me to your mailing list. My principal interests are:

....

Name: ....
(Block letters please)
Address: ....

....

Postcode: ....

Neil Poppmacher
BMJ Publishing Group
BMA House
Tavistock Square
LONDON
WC1H 9BR

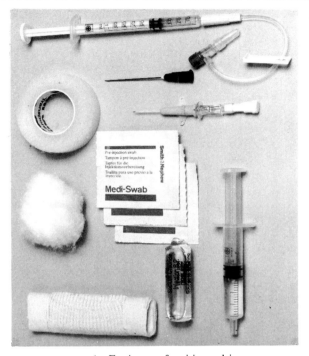

FIG 1   Equipment for siting a drip

heparinised saline and attached to a T connector is useful to keep the cannula patent while the giving set is prepared.

Preparation of the child

A young child should be held by a parent where possible (Fig 2). Select a suitable vein on the hand, arm, or foot. If time allows, apply local anaesthetic cream (EMLA cream 5%) to one or two suitable veins 60 minutes beforehand. When ready, the child should be held sideways on the mother's lap with one arm behind her back. The mother will be responsible for holding the child's trunk and, if she wishes, screening the child's view with her free hand. A nurse will hold the drip hand or foot braced against the mother's knee. Explain to the child that you are going to "make a scratch on his hand which will hurt for a moment, and then put a big bandage on it". A small baby may be swaddled tightly in a

31

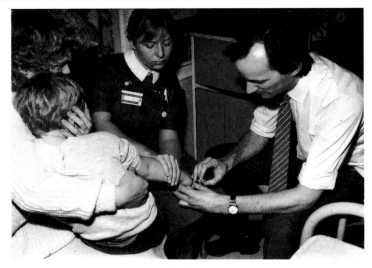

FIG 2   Holding the patient

sheet, leaving the chosen limb free, and held by the nurse. Scalp
veins in the parietal or temporal region may be chosen, in which
case some of the hair will need to be shaved using a disposable
razor.

Insertion of the cannula

Ideal veins for cannulation are those that are easily immobilised
– for example, the median cubital vein, which is fixed in fascia, or a
vein on the hand with a Y junction, which prevents the vein from
moving away during insertion of the needle (Fig 3). Ensure that
the vein is well filled with blood, if necessary by a peristaltic
pumping action from above. The assistant must not squeeze so
hard as to cut off the arterial supply. Swab the skin well with
alcohol and allow to dry. Pierce the skin about 5 mm from the point
at which the vein will be entered, using a separate needle, as the
fine plastic cannula is easily damaged. Pass the cannula on its
needle through the same hole in the skin and lift the tip of the
needle so that it is moving superficially in the subcutaneous layer.
Aim to enter the vein from above, preferably in the angle of the Y
junction. Once the needle is in the lumen and blood is seen flashing

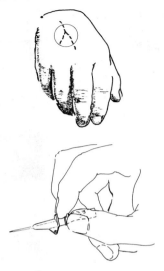

FIG 3   Insert the cannula into a Y junction. When blood flushes back, push the cannula forward with the forefinger

back from the needle hub, lift up the bevel of the needle and advance it until the cannula itself is in the lumen of the vein. Most cannulas now have a raised shoulder at the hub which can be pressed gently with the forefinger to hold the cannula stationary in the lumen of the vein while the needle is withdrawn. If this process has been successfully accomplished blood will be seen flushing back up the cannula as the needle is withdrawn. If no blood flushes back it is likely that the vein has been transfixed and that the cannula tip is below the vein. Remove the needle completely and pull back the cannula slowly until blood flushes back. Lay the cannula hub as flat as possible on the skin and advance the cannula into the lumen of the vein.

When the cannula is in the lumen attach the 1 ml syringe and inject a little saline. Keep flushing saline slowly into the vein and gently push the cannula through the skin up to the hub.

Securing the cannula (Fig 4)

Clean away any spilt blood from the skin and cannula using a spirit swab and allow to dry. Place a strip of tape under the wings

(a)

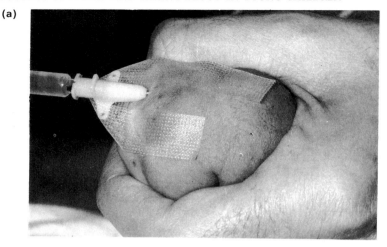

(b)

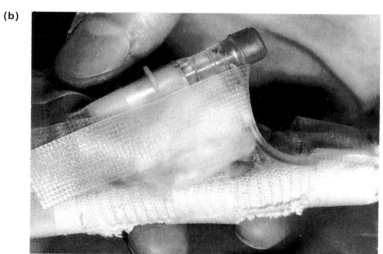

FIG 4   Securing the cannula

of the cannula adhesive side up, and fold the tape over the wings and stick it parallel to the line of the cannula. Put a further strip of tape over the hub of the cannula. Replace the 1 ml syringe with the T connector. Strap the hand or arm gently to the splint. Try to avoid putting tape circumferentially around the arm proximal to

34

the catheter tip as this will impede flow from the cannula and encourage thrombophlebitis. Insert some cotton wool behind the hub of the cannula and strap gently. Tape the T connector firmly to the splint.

If potentially irritant fluids containing calcium salts, amino acids, or some drugs are infused, serious necrosis of the skin can follow extravasation. An intravenous site should be inspected every hour without removing any adhesive by the nurse looking after the infant. Increasing swelling or redness should be investigated and the infusion stopped if extravasation is suspected.

Inspect the intravenous site every hour

Scalp vein infusion with butterfly needle

Explain to the mother that the needle is not going inside the skull, the needle is painless after insertion, and the hair will grow back. Shave the hair on the temporoparietal area on one side. Palpate the vessel and check the direction of blood flow to ensure that a vein and not an artery will be infused. Avoid the forehead because extravasation of irritant solutions may leave a scar. Immobilise all but the smallest infants by wrapping in a sheet.

Prepare the butterfly needle (short 25 or 23 gauge) by filling it with 0·9% saline. Cut strips of narrow adhesive and gauze impregnated with plaster of Paris. Make a tourniquet with an elastic band around the head or a finger proximal to the site of insertion. Select a Y junction or straight vein and insert the needle 0·5 cm away from the planned point of entry as this will help to stabilise the needle. Insert the needle into the vein from above and see that blood will flow back along the tubing. Inject some saline and check for subcutaneous swelling. Tape down the wings of the needle and pack a little cotton wool or plaster of Paris behind the needle to keep the butterfly needle at the optimum angle for infusion. Plaster of Paris may be spread over the wings giving effective immobilisation. The needle should remain visible to detect extravasation. A plastic cup with two sections cut out gives protection while providing visibility (Fig 5).

35

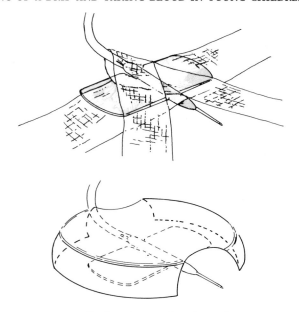

FIG 5   Securing a scalp vein needle

Emergency vascular access

Even a skilled paediatrician may find it difficult to site a drip in a moribund, hypovolaemic infant. Remember that some emergency drugs, such as 1 : 10 000 adrenaline, atropine, and naloxone, can be given via an endotracheal tube in an emergency. Internal jugular puncture or subclavian puncture should only be attempted by those skilled in their use. The external jugular vein or scalp veins may prove accessible if the child is held in a head down position. The bone marrow provides a convenient route for the administration of drugs, fluid, and blood: an intraosseous infusion needle or a wide bore butterfly needle should be inserted into the bone marrow of the tibia 1–3 cm below the tibial tuberosity after careful skin preparation. Strong hypertonic solutions such as 50% dextrose or 10% calcium gluconate should of course be avoided, but otherwise this route to the circulation is suitable for a wide range of dextrose–electrolyte solutions, plasma, blood, and drugs.[1]

Taking blood

Venepuncture

Blood samples may readily be obtained using a 23 gauge butterfly needle and syringe, adopting the above technique. Use the smallest possible syringe so that you can aspirate very gently, otherwise the vein will collapse. If the blood is required for culture sterilise the skin with povidine–iodine solution and allow to dry.

Blood may be obtained from small babies by allowing it to drip directly from the needle into the sampling bottles. Use a wide bore needle (for example, 21 gauge) and break off the hub before inserting the needle into the vein. If the baby's hand is held in the operator's palm with the fingers flexed blood can be "pumped" into the baby's hand by a peristaltic action. This technique is not suitable for obtaining blood for culture.

Capillary blood sampling

In babies under six months old, the heel is the ideal site for capillary blood sampling, but in older infants the thumb is better. The heel must be warm: if it is cold dip the foot into hand warm water (40°C) for five minutes and then dry it thoroughly. Hold the foot by encircling the ball of the heel with your thumb and forefinger. Select a site on the side of the heel, wipe it with isopropyl alcohol, and allow to dry. Do not use the ball or back of the heel because a painful ulcer may form. Apply a thin layer of soft paraffin to the chosen site so that the blood will not smear during sampling. Insert a disposable lancet about 2 mm and withdraw, cutting very slightly sideways. Wipe away the initial drop of blood with a dry cotton swab and then let the drops form and fall into the container. Squeeze and release your fingers around the calf to milk blood into the heel. Agitate the container to mix the blood with anticoagulant. When the required volume has been obtained wipe the heel and press with a clean cotton wool ball. This method is not suitable for obtaining blood for culture or for coagulation studies.

Gloves should be worn for all procedures involving blood

Always wear rubber gloves when taking blood or siting a drip, to minimise the risk of acquiring blood borne disease, such as hepatitis or human immunodeficiency virus.

Reference

Orlowski JP. My kingdom for an intravenous line. *Am J Dis Child* 1984; **138:** 803.

4 Arterial puncture

AN THOMAS

Obtaining an arterial blood gas sample is an essential step in the assessment of any patient with respiratory failure or critical illness. The presence of abnormal physical findings – for example, changes in respiratory rate, breathing pattern, cyanosis, or evidence of hypoperfusion – indicates the patients from whom an arterial blood gas sample should be obtained.

The correct interpretation of the blood gas results enables us to make a quantitative judgement about the degree of cardiorespiratory derangement. Blood gas analysis also points to possible causes or derangement and will help in monitoring the response to treatment.

Indications

The main indication for arterial puncture is the need for arterial blood for blood gas analysis. Arterial puncture is also rarely indicated where it has proved impossible to obtain a venous blood sample for other investigations.

Contraindications

There are no absolute contraindications to arterial puncture.

Site of puncture

The commonly used sites for arterial puncture are the brachial, radial, and femoral arteries. Choice of the most suitable site for a particular patient will be guided by the clinical situation (Box A) and by operator preference. It is wise to perform a radial or brachial artery puncture on the patient's non-dominant arm.

Box A   Indications and contraindications, advantages and disadvantages of the commonly used sites for arterial puncture

Radial artery

Indications and advantages
- Easily accessible
- Easily compressible, therefore useful if there is a known bleeding tendency

Contraindications and disadvantages
- Buerger's disease
- Raynaud's disease
- Arteriovenous dialysis shunt present or imminent
- Absent ulnar collateral circulation
- Venous sample may be obtained

Brachial artery

Indications and advantages
- Easily accessible

Contraindications and disadvantages
- Arteriovenous fistula in arm
- Elbow fractures
- End artery, therefore theoretical risk of ischaemia
- Venous sample may be obtained

Femoral artery

Indications and advantages
- May be the only quickly accessible artery in the shocked patient

Contraindications and disadvantages
- Severe peripheral vascular disease
- Aortofemoral bypass surgery
- Venous sample more likely than other sites

Procedure

Before proceeding with arterial puncture it is important that you and the patient are properly prepared (Box B and table) and that you have the appropriate equipment (Box C).

Once you are satisfied with your preparations you may proceed. Although the basic principles of arterial puncture are similar for all three commonly used sites, there are some important differences between the sites; these differences are summarised in the table.

Box B   Preparations before arterial puncture

- Explain the procedure to patient and obtain consent
- Make arrangements with laboratory/ICU/portering staff for immediate analysis of sample before obtaining it
- If blood gas analysis is not going to be performed within a few minutes have an ice bag ready to cool the sample
- Note type of oxygen therapy and check whether the patient is getting the oxygen you think he or she is. (Is the flowmeter turned on? Is the tubing correctly connected? If a Venti-mask is used is the oxygen flow appropriate for that mask?)
- Check that the oxygen concentration has remained constant for at least 15 minutes before sampling. (Has the patient kept his or her mask on?)
- The help of an assistant is very useful when performing an arterial puncture
- Position the patient
- Wear disposable gloves and make sure the assistant does the same. Make sure a sharps bin is available close at hand

---

Box C   Equipment required for arterial puncture

- Non-sterile disposable gloves for doctor and assistant
- Alcohol swabs or other antiseptic solution
- Syringe of *plain* lignocaine and gauge 25 or 27 needle
- Blood gas syringe with gauge 23 needle (if not available normal 2 ml syringe may be used)
- Heparin 1000 units/ml if not in blood gas syringe
- Cotton wool balls to press over site after arterial puncture

Differences in technique between puncture sites

Puncture site	Positioning of patient	Angle of needle to skin (°)	Puncture site	Important anatomical structures in proximity to puncture site
Femoral	Supine	60	Mid inguinal point 2 cm below inguinal ligament	Femoral vein medial Femoral nerve lateral
Brachial	Arm extended and supported on pillow	30	Medial to biceps tendon in antecubital fossa	Median nerve medial
Radial	Arm extended and supported on pillow with wrist extended 20°	30	Proximal to proximal transverse crease lateral aspect of wrist	

Once the site has been selected the area is cleaned and the gas syringe primed with heparin. If a normal 2 ml syringe is used, about 0·25 ml heparin 1000 units/ml is drawn into the syringe. The plunger is then pulled back to coat the walls of the syringe with heparin, after which the syringe is emptied to leave only a small amount of heparin in the bevel of the syringe and the needle. If a special blood gas syringe is used (for example, Pulsator from Concord Laboratories, Kent), then the syringe will already contain either heparin or heparin in solution. Excess solution should be expelled as above. These special syringes have the advantage of producing low friction between the wall and the plunger, and will therefore fill under the pressure of arterial, but not venous, blood without the operator having to pull on the plunger.

Then 0·5–1 ml 1% plain lignocaine is infiltrated under the skin and adjacent to the artery.

Always aspirate before injection of local anaesthetics. Use of local anaesthesia in the conscious patient is essential because arterial puncture is painful.

Never use adrenaline containing solutions because these may cause vessel spasm and ischaemia

---

The artery should now be palpated carefully. To overcome the loss of sensitivity caused by wearing gloves, three fingers should be used to palpate the artery (Fig 1). These should be placed at several points, moving medially to laterally over the course of the artery to determine the point of maximum pulsation. Once the artery has been located the gauge 23 needle of the blood gas syringe is advanced, bevel up, towards the artery (Fig 2). With experience, the pulsation of the artery can be felt through the syringe just before arterial puncture. If a special blood gas syringe is used, the low resistance between the plunger and the syringe wall allows blood to pulsate into the syringe, so confirming arterial puncture. If a normal syringe is used gentle traction is needed to draw blood into the syringe.

Arteries tend to be in close proximity to nerves and if, during attempted puncture, the patient complains of sharp shooting pains then it must be assumed that the needle has entered the nerve. The needle should be removed and redirected.

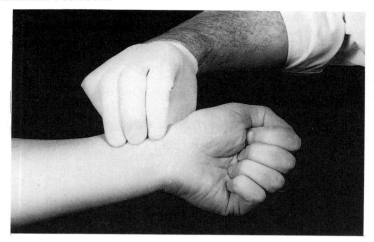

FIG 1   Positioning of fingers to obtain arterial pulse

If no blood is obtained after the needle has been advanced for an appropriate distance, withdraw the needle slowly with gentle traction on the plunger. Arterial blood will often enter the syringe during its removal. If this does not happen redirect the needle and try again. Repeated unsuccessful attempts are painful to the

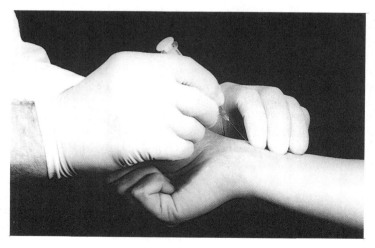

FIG 2   Needle positioning for radial artery puncture

patient and may delay urgent therapeutic manoeuvres so you will need to get help in this situation.

After 1·5–2 ml blood have been obtained the needle and syringe should be removed and the assistant should press firmly on the puncture site for five minutes. After this time the site should be inspected and if there is evidence of continued bleeding then pressure should be reapplied until it stops. The needle should be disconnected from the syringe and dropped in the adjacent sharps bin.

> **Never re-sheath a needle, and never pass the needle or needle and syringe to an assistant**

Any bubbles in the syringe should be gently removed by holding the syringe bevel up, and tapping the syringe to allow bubbles to pass into the bevel. They can then be flushed out into a cotton wool ball held over the tip of the syringe. A cap should then be placed over the bevel and the sample sent for analysis (Fig 3). An accompanying laboratory request form should state the inspired

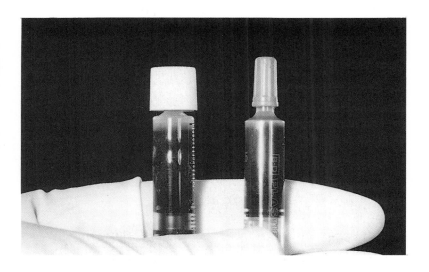

FIG 3   Capped syringes posing no threat of needlestick injury

45

oxygen concentration (21% if room air). This allows calculation of the arterial–alveolar oxygen gradient by the blood gas analyser and provides essential information for anyone attempting to interpret the blood gas results.

5 Urethral and suprapubic catheterisation

NJR GEORGE

Instrumentation of the urinary bladder is one of the oldest described surgical procedures; however, in only a few is the future health of the patient so threatened by the consequences of poor or inappropriate technique. A clear understanding of the indications for, and the complications of, bladder drainage, as well as an appreciation of anatomical and bacteriological detail, is essential before catheterisation can take place.

Indications for catheterisation

> **Indications**
> - Pain
> - Obstructive renal failure
> - Incontinence
> - Pelvic trauma

There are three fundamental reasons for catheter drainage of urine: pain, obstructive renal failure, and disabling incontinence. To these a fourth, relatively rare indication may be added: catheterisation as part of the management of severe pelvic trauma. If none of these indications is present, the clinician must seriously question why the procedure is being undertaken.

Pain

The pain of acute urinary retention is exquisite and will probably be the patient's worst experience to date. Classically the "£100 test" ("Would you give £100 to be relieved of the pain by catheterisation?") is answered without hesitation in the affirmative. Cases with other semi-intense dysuria or perineal discomfort caused by acute cystitis or prostatitis never evoke this response; in these patients the lack of lower abdominal swelling (dull to percussion, no lower margin) on mandatory abdominal examination will confirm the absence of retention.

Obstructive renal failure

Upper tract dilatation with possible compromise of renal function is only found in about 5% of patients with classic bladder outflow tract obstruction caused by benign prostatic hypertrophy; therefore the typical patient presenting in casualty with a painful distended bladder is unlikely to have postrenal obstructive failure. By contrast, patients with an enlarged (often grossly so) *painless* bladder may frequently demonstrate renal impairment; in such cases a request for emergency biochemistry is essential, although catheterisation is only required if urinary creatinine is elevated. The advice of a urologist is essential under these circumstances because unnecessary catheterisation of the distended painless bladder may prejudice the patient's subsequent clinical management (see below). Most urologists will accept a serum creatinine level in the range 200–250 μmol/l if an operation can be scheduled within days; above this level preoperative intervention is usually required.

Incontinence

Catheterisation is decreasing as a management choice in patients with incontinence, partly as a result of newer surgical techniques in the old and infirm, and partly as a result of improved nursing management in the elderly. Nevertheless, severe urinary incontinence which soaks the patient, his or her bed, and clothes remains an indication for controlled drainage if only to afford relief for both the individual and those attempting to manage the situation.

48

Urethral injury – pelvic trauma

Severe pelvic trauma which disrupts the osseous ring and local crush (astride) injuries in the region of the urogenital diaphragm may cause variable damage to the urethra, ranging from mild bruising to complete disruption and dislocation of the bladder or sphincter mechanism. If there is any suggestion of such urethral injury – blood at meatus, severe perineal bruising, distended bladder with difficulty initiating micturition, or "absent" prostate on rectal examination, which implies upward displacement of the bladder – urethral catheterisation must *not* be attempted and the advice of a urologist should be urgently sought. Under these circumstances it is likely that suprapubic catheterisation will be required. Further iatrogenic urethral trauma, with almost certain introduction of organisms into the haematoma, can rapidly convert a lesion capable of healing into one requiring extensive and prolonged reconstructive surgery.

Warning – in pelvic trauma

- Blood at meatus
- Severe perineal bruising
- Distended bladder and difficulty in initiating micturition
- "Absent" prostate on rectal examination

Do not attempt urethral catheterisation

Penalties of catheterisation

Penalties

- Local trauma
- Infection
- Discomfort
- Erosion
- Bypassing
- Bladder shrinkage

Local trauma

In inexperienced hands the urethral catheter is both a painful and a dangerous weapon. Even knowledge of the local anatomy (see below) may not ensure against damage, particularly in the bulbar region, if the wrong type of catheter is selected; application of inappropriate pressure can lead to false passage and subsequent stricture formation.

Infection

Although organisms may be introduced at the time of catheterisation with an inadequate technique, it is well known that even ideal placement can eventually lead to infection of the lower urinary tract. In these circumstances the organisms are known to ascend between the catheter and the urethral wall; bladder urine will be colonised, on average, three days after urethral and five days after suprapubic catheterisation. For this reason patients presenting with acute retention require prophylactic preoperative antibiotics if their prostate operation cannot be performed at short notice after admission.

Discomfort

A urethral catheter and its attachments are very uncomfortable for the patient, particularly if made of any sort of plastic. Although most catheters are pliable at body temperature, they become stiff at the meatus which often leads to considerable soreness. The attachments of the catheter bag should be adjusted to reduce such discomfort to a minimum, taking into account the patient's usual posture.

Erosion

The urethra is, in effect, "shut" at rest and the presence of an oversized catheter may sometimes cause pressure ulceration of the wall. Typically, patients with incontinence and bypassing are catheterised with catheters of ever larger diameter; this almost never works and can eventually lead to mucosal erosion (Fig 1).

Bypassing

The presence of a balloon on the trigone leads to bladder spasms in most patients; these often give rise to paracatheter leakage of urine (bypassing) and sharp lower abdominal cramp-like pains. The balloon of the catheter should be inflated to the minimum practical volume to ensure retention; however, this distressing symptom is usually only relieved following removal of the tube.

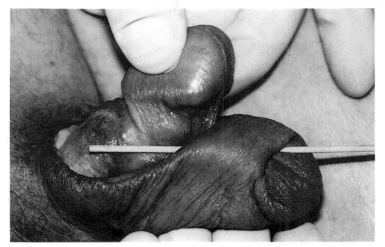

FIG 1   A combination of impaired sensation and an over-large catheter inserted for incontinence led to gross urethral (not seen) and penile skin ulceration in this diabetic patient

Bladder shrinkage

Typically, the tense painless bladder of chronic retention (frequently associated with obstructive uropathy) may experience significant shrinking after catheterisation, often to volumes of 200–300 ml. Such small volumes may make for difficult transurethral resection; preoperative catheterisation is thus best avoided in such cases unless significant renal impairment (see above) is present.

Catheter construction

The material strength of the catheter wall determines the maximal luminal cross-section which can be supported without collapse of the drainage tube (Fig 2). Traditionally catheter measurement is by the external circumference of the tube in millimetres (known as Charrière (Ch) or French gauge). Hence, size for size, a stiff plastic catheter will allow a larger drainage channel (at the cost of patient discomfort) than a soft, but necessarily thick walled, latex catheter. Silicone, which is also soft but non-reactive for long term usage, tends to be thicker walled with consequent smaller lumen. Hence plastic catheters are ideal for

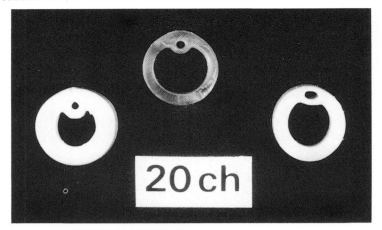

FIG 2   Material wall strength of (left to right) latex, plastic, and silicone catheters determines the cross-sectional area of the drainage channel in any one size of catheter

drainage of debris or blood (that is, postoperative) from the bladder whereas latex and silicone catheters are used regularly for short (<one week) and long (8–10 weeks) term drainage of clear urine. Latex, although cheap and comfortable for the patient, is unsuitable for long term drainage because urine reacts with constituents in the rubber precipitating material which rapidly blocks the lumen. Earlier problems with cytotoxicity of this material have been overcome.

Types of catheter

Various types of catheter are available which assist drainage under differing circumstances (Fig 3). Opposed eye catheters are the most common type whereas whistle tip catheters are open at the distal end – the most effective design for evacuation of solid debris, blood clot, etc, from the bladder. The bend at the distal end of a Coudé (French elbow) catheter is extremely useful to help guide the tube around the bend in the bulbar region of the male urethra. Most catheters found in wards or accident departments will have Foley balloons and an associated inflation channel for self-retention. A third channel, which marginally narrows the bore of the main drainage lumen, is present in irrigating catheters used to wash out the lower urinary tract.

(a)

(b)

(c)

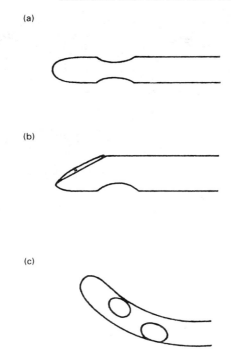

FIG 3   Common types of catheter: (a) opposed eye, (b) open ended "whistle tip", and (c) Coudé

Types of catheter

- Opposed eye catheters
- Whistle tip catheters
- Coudé catheters
- Suprapubic catheters

Despite this wide choice, the typical patient presenting in retention will almost invariably be best served by urethral passage of a 16 or 18 Ch Coudé plastic catheter with Foley balloon. Sizes below 12 Ch are usually too pliable to be clinically useful in the general ward or emergency setting whereas 22 and 24 Ch catheters (sizes proceed in even numbers) are almost exclusively for use in the operative and postoperative situation.

Suprapubic catheters are of smaller size, usually between 10 and 14 Ch and most are introduced by either a sharp internal metal or plastic obturator, or an external sheath which can be removed easily after insertion (Fig 4). The catheters are retained by either the Foley balloon technique or a variety of mechanisms including pig tail memory or simple suture of a flange to the surface of the abdominal wall.

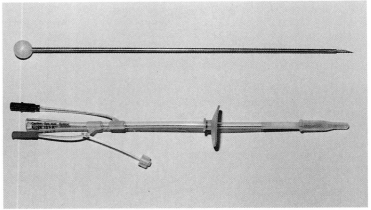

FIG 4   Typical suprapubic catheter with internal steel stylette, tip guarded by a plastic sheath, Foley retention balloon with inflation side arm, flange for skin suture, and urine sampling port

Anatomical essentials

Male urethra

Sympathetic catheterisation of the male is not possible without a working knowledge of the anatomy of the urethra and associated mechanisms (Fig 5). By holding it straight during the catheterisation procedure (see below), the penile urethra passes directly to the bulbar region where a smooth bend of almost 90° occurs leading directly to the sphincter mechanism. The subsequent prostatic urethra is of variable length depending on the size of the gland. Extensive sensory nerves supply the mucosal lining of the urethra; dilatation of the sphincter as the catheter passes through causes an acute sensation of impending micturition which passes after a short interval with the tube in situ.

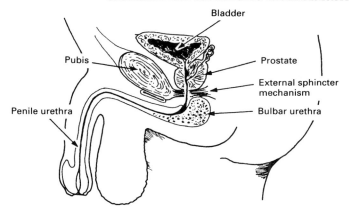

FIG 5   Anatomy of the male urethra

Female urethra

Localisation of the female urethra is usually not difficult (behind the clitoris) and the sensation of sphincter dilatation is identical to that experienced by the male. Occasionally previous continence surgery (ie, colposuspension) may draw up the urethra into an "intravaginal" position; catheterisation under these circumstances may be surprisingly difficult.

Suprapubic anatomy

Appreciation of the layers through which a suprapubic catheter must pass is important if the technique is to be successful (Fig 6a). Three tough barriers – the skin, linea alba, and detrusor muscle – must be cleanly penetrated during introduction of the drainage tube. The enlarging bladder lifts the peritoneum off the posterior aspect of the abdominal wall; a volume of 300 ml is required before this is palpable suprapubically. In a typical patient, it is unlikely that a catheter could be introduced with confidence, using a suprapubic approach, into a bladder containing less than 500 ml (Fig 6b).

(a)

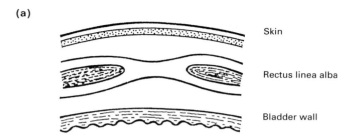

Skin

Rectus linea alba

Bladder wall

(b)

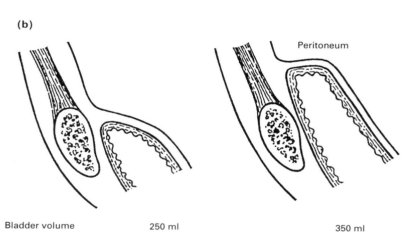

Peritoneum

Bladder volume   250 ml   350 ml

FIG 6   (a) Important layers in the suprapubic approach to the bladder. (b) Peritoneum and bowel displaced from the anterior abdominal wall as the bladder enlarges

Technique of catheterisation

Trolley lay-up

Introduction of bacteria into the lower urinary tract may have serious consequences and every effort must be made to ensure that catheterisation is a completely sterile procedure. These days it can be assumed that no assistance will be available and the trolley will be prepared accordingly without omitting any of the items listed (Box A) on the bottom level; the top is cleaned with antiseptic in the approved manner (see Appendix).

Box A   Requirements for sterile trolley

Catheter pack	Waterproof paper
	Paper towel
	Kidney dish
	Galley pots
	Gauze swabs
	Plastic forceps
Additions	Aqueous chlorhexidine
	Sterile lignocaine gel + nozzle
	20 ml syringe/sterile water
	Catheter
	Catheter bag with tubing
	Gloves

Approach to patient

Nothing is more alarming to a patient than the approach of a doctor whose intention is to operate in the perineal region. A sympathetic explanation of what is about to happen and the precautions to be taken against pain are essential. To state that the procedure will not hurt is misleading; it is better to explain that the introduction of the catheter "will just feel like passing water" which lowers both anxiety and tension in the pelvic floor and permits easier passage into the bladder.

Catheterisation of the male

Assuming the operator is right handed, ensure that adequate access is available on the right side of the patient for both doctor and dressing trolley. The patient should be reclining but not flat – the latter position increases the pain of acute retention considerably. Remove the patient's trousers and underclothes so that the legs may be parted easily to accommodate the kidney dish.

Lay out the top of the trolley, making sure all items required are opened and accessible. Having washed, don sterile gloves and, with a gauze swab, grasp the distal shaft of the penis, thoroughly cleansing the glans with further swabs soaked in aqeous chlorhexidine. Continue to hold the distal penis away from the scrotum while inserting the large waterproof paper between the legs and up under the penile shaft which may then be laid on the sterile paper.

Taking the tube of sterile anaesthetic gel (1–2% lignocaine), elevate the penile shaft and gently – pain is caused by urethral distension – express the contents explaining what is happening to the patient. Passage of gel to the bulb may be encouraged by suitable backward massage of the corpus spongiosus; soft penile clamps, once available to retain the gel, are infrequently found in catheter packs nowadays.

Having allowed about five minutes for the anaesthetic to work, again elevate and straighten the penile urethra. Place the kidney dish in readiness on the waterproof sheet between the thighs. Ideally the "no touch" technique should be used in which the operator has no contact with the catheter shaft (sterile gloves included); disposable plastic forceps are usually provided in catheter packs for this purpose. Typically a 16 or 18 Ch Coudé catheter will have been selected, and this is grasped in the plastic forceps taking care to ensure that the direction of the elbow bend (usually the same axis as the catheter side arm) is pointing upwards. Slide the tube gently down the straightened penile urethra and pause at the bulb. Tell the patient it is about to "slide round the bend" and pause again outside the sphincter. Inform the patient that he will feel as if he is about to pass water, ask him again to relax, and slowly push the catheter into the bladder at which point urine should issue and fall into the kidney dish. Push the catheter in almost to the side arm before inflating the Foley balloon with sterile water. Once connected, it is sound bacteriological practice not to disconnect the drainage bag unless absolutely necessary. Record the volume of urine drained in the patient's notes and send a specimen for bacteriological examination.

Warning

- After catheter insertion ensure the foreskin (if present) is replaced over the glans

---

Troubleshooting

Paradoxically, the sphincter muscles in patients with acute retention are relaxed by reflex action and passage of a catheter is surprisingly easy. If the catheter will not pass any part of the urethra with gentle pressure, or if a trace of blood is seen on the catheter tip on withdrawal, do *not* persevere or push harder as serious damage may ensue. Senior assistance will be required in this event. Never blow up the Foley balloon if doubt exists about whether it has entered the bladder; pain on inflation may indicate that severe iatrogenic trauma is taking place. A catheter introducer, which can cause devastating damage, should never be used except by the most experienced.

Warning
- Catheter will not pass with gentle pressure
- Blood on catheter when withdrawn

Seek Senior help

Occasionally the foreskin may be so tight as to obscure the lumen in the glans. Under these circumstances, extra lignocaine gel injected into the space under the foreskin will distend it slightly, allowing the phimotic meatus and true meatus to align with one another; the catheter then almost invariably passes successfully directly across the space into the urethral lumen.

Catheterisation of the female

The comparatively simple anatomy of females ensures that there are usually few problems associated with this procedure. The semi-lithotomy position of thighs apart with flexed knees is best adopted; during cleansing and introduction of the catheter the labia are conveniently held apart by the thumb and index finger of the left hand, thus avoiding perineal contamination of the catheter shaft. Although some omit lignocaine gel for female catheterisation, this is helpful to the patient, particularly for the lubricant value of the material.

Suprapubic catheterisation

For obvious reasons, introduction of a suprapubic catheter is a more "surgical" approach to bladder drainage than the urethral method and as such is less familiar to most junior doctors. Nevertheless, as stated above, it has significant advantages includ-

59

ing a lesser risk of bacteriological contamination, greater patient comfort, and absence of potential urethral trauma.

The clinician must of course be *completely confident* that the bladder is enlarged suprapubically. Apart from eliciting the typical physical signs (see above) it is mandatory to obtain urine by aspiration with a "green" (21 gauge) needle and syringe before proceeding. A small bleb of local anaesthetic is placed in the midline about 4 cm above the pubic symphysis and the needle passed sharply downwards and slightly caudally to the hilt before aspirating to confirm that urine is present.

Following confirmation of the enlarged bladder, the skin and structures down to and including the bladder wall are infiltrated with 2% lignocaine, carefully explaining to the patient what is being done while proceeding slowly and so giving the anaesthetic time to work (approximately five minutes). The skin of the lower abdomen is now cleansed and the area above the umbilicus and below the pubis masked off with the paper or cloth towels provided in the suprapubic catheter pack. The three tough layers (see above) have to be penetrated and, to avoid unnecessary pushing (which is very alarming for the patient), the skin and linea alba (rectus sheath) should be adequately punctured with a no. 11 scalpel blade. The suprapubic catheter is then passed along the track, downwards and caudally, and steady controlled pressure exerted until it enters the bladder. In a muscular man this pressure, which exacerbates the patient's desire to urinate if he is in acute retention, may need to be surprisingly firm yet controlled and is the cause of much of the anxiety experienced by doctors attempting the technique for the first time.

The most common error when performing this technique is to cease pushing before the catheter and balloon are fully within the bladder lumen. After the firm resistance of the rectus sheath, the tip of the catheter will enter the bladder and urine will be observed to well out; the balloon, however, has yet to pass through the third resistance layer (the detrusor wall) and, unless continued pressure is applied to attain this objective, the balloon will be blown up in the extraperitoneal space. Urine drains for a while and then stops as the bladder falls away from the tip of the catheter. If this has happened it will be necessary to wait until the bladder refills to a degree; then it is safe to attempt a further passage of the tube. Depending on catheter type, the shaft may be stitched to the skin for additional confidence and the whole covered with a dressing to prevent snagging on the patient's clothes.

Aftercare and complications

Complications
- Pain at meatal tip
- Kinking of tube to drainage bag
- Postobstructive diuresis
- Infections
- Decompression of Foley balloon

Pain at meatal tip

This discomfort has been mentioned earlier. Some relief may be obtained if a gauze swab is wrapped around the catheter as it emerges; if moistened with an antiseptic solution, it may also provide a useful antibacterial barrier to ascending organisms.

Drainage bag

Ensure that the patient understands that the bag must be below the level of his or her bladder and the tube placed through the metal "eye" on the catheter stand to prevent kinking and blockage.

Postobstructive diuresis

Patients with chronic retention and obstructive uropathy may have a brisk postobstructive diuresis following bladder catheterisation; this is related to impaired distal tubular function. A description of the duration and management of this important physiological abnormality is beyond the scope of this text; however, it should be noted that it is unusual for the patient to require intravenous replacement therapy. In most cases the urine usually becomes blood stained (often heavily so) about 10–15 minutes after catheterisation and this is the result of mucosal bleeding from both upper and lower tracts; it is not traumatic catheterisation as is sometimes thought. The bleeding settles within 24–36 hours and the urine clears.

Long term catheterisation and infection

It is inevitable that patients with long term silicone catheters will have infected urine caused by the presence of the foreign body within the bladder. Unless the patient has been on antibiotics for other reasons the organisms are usually of low grade and require no treatment – indeed misguided antibiotic therapy usually allows the emergence of virulent strains which can be difficult to eradicate. Occasionally the presence of low grade organisms within the bladder may cause a temporary bacteraemia (catheter fever) when the old catheter is changed. If this is the case, a single shot before the tube change of a suitable antibiotic against Gram-negative organisms will usually prevent the complication.

Foley balloon decompression

Occasionally Foley balloons may fail to decompress because of a fault in the balloon channel or encrustation around the catheter tip if it has been in situ for too long. Passage of a fine wire (ie, guidewire of an ureteric catheter) down the balloon channel (having first cut off the Luer valve) may resolve the situation. Injection down the channel of any chemicals that are latex solvents is no longer advised. In the male if all else fails ultrasonically guided suprapubic needle puncture may be required. In the female a needle may be introduced with great care between the urethral wall and the catheter shaft and, guided by a finger in the vagina, the balloon can be punctured easily.

6 Central venous cannulation

M ROSEN
IP LATTO
W SHANG NG

Central venous cannulation has become one of the most commonly practised procedures. The procedure may, however, result in serious hazard and even death. There are numerous approaches to the central veins, and the methods and equipment described here have been chosen as those most likely to be safe and successful in the hands of a junior doctor called on to cannulate an adult.

Indications and contraindications

Central venous pressure is the resultant of venous blood volume, right ventricular function, and venous tone. Rapid changes in blood volume, especially associated with impaired right heart function, are the most common reason for monitoring central venous pressure (Fig 1). Pressures measured in peripheral veins cannot be relied on to reflect these changes. Infusions of antibiotics, chemotherapeutic agents, and other substances irritant to veins and tissues are best administered through a line whose tip lies in a central vein. Potent drugs such as catecholamine solutions given at very slow flow rates are most reliably given through a central venous line. Drugs used in resuscitation of cardiac arrest should be given through a central line if one is available. In an emergency only a central vein may be accessible for administration of a rapid lifesaving infusion. A central venous line is also widely used for long term intravenous alimentation. More sophisticated indications for central venous access include the insertion of a Swan–Ganz catheter and intracardiac pacing devices.

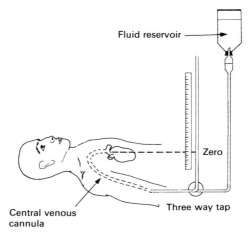

FIG 1   Measuring central venous pressure

Indications for central venous cannulation

- Monitor central venous pressure
- Irritant infusion administration
- Catecholamine infusion
- Drug administration in cardiac arrest
- Swan–Ganz catheter and transvenous pacing

There are no absolute contraindications to the method per se. Venepuncture should be avoided, however, at any site at which there is sepsis. Apical emphysema or bullae contraindicate infra-clavicular or supraclavicular approaches to the subclavian vein. A carotid artery aneurysm precludes using the internal jugular vein on the same side. Furthermore, it may be wise to reconsider central venous cannulation in hypocoagulation and hypercoagulation states or if there is septicaemia.

Procedure

Sterility

Sterility should be maintained during the insertion of the

cannula. The skin should be carefully cleaned – for example, with 0·5% chlorhexidine in 70% alcohol – and sterile towels applied round the site. The operator should wear a mask, gown, and gloves. In an emergency gloves at least should be worn. Although some catheter systems are designed to be used ungloved, in practice contamination may sometimes occur through an error or technical difficulty. A syringe filled with heparinised saline (heparin 10 units/ml in physiological saline) is useful for flushing the line as soon as it is inserted.

Equipment (Fig 2)
Catheter through cannula

This type of device is recommended for inserting a long catheter through an arm vein. A well designed example is the New Drum Cartridge Catheter. A cannula on the outside of a needle is placed in the vein and the needle withdrawn. A catheter is inserted through the cannula and is then threaded into the vein. When the catheter is in position the cannula is withdrawn.

Catheter over needle

In an arm vein the needle and the catheter are placed in the vein, the needle (which is attached to a wire) withdrawn, and the catheter advanced into position. A shorter version of this is the long cannula over a long needle (100–150 mm) which is intended for use in the internal jugular and subclavian veins. A safety

Diameters of needles or cannulas and lengths of catheters recommended for each route of insertion

Route of insertion	Outside diameter of needle or cannula (gauge)	Minimum length of catheter (mm)
Arm vein	14	600
External jugular vein	16 or 14	200
Internal jugular vein	16 or 14	150*
Subclavian vein	16 or 14	150*

* Long cannulas are available (120–150 mm long, 14–18 gauge outside diameter).

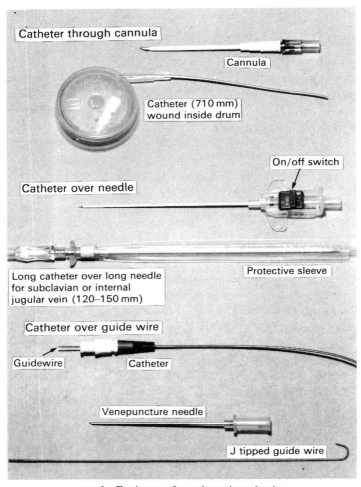

FIG 2   Equipment for catheter introduction

feature in some of these devices is a means of occluding the hub to prevent bleeding and air embolism – Wallace Flexihub, Secalon T.

Catheter through needle

This is the simplest method and was once widely used. It has been condemned because improper use may result in the catheter being sheared off. Most manufacturers have withdrawn this type of apparatus.

Catheter over guide wire

A flexible guide wire is inserted into the vein through a small gauge needle. After removal of the needle the catheter is inserted over the wire, which guides it into the vein. This technique is recommended as a safer alternative to the long cannula on long needle method for internal jugular and subclavian vein catheterisation because probing for the vein is carried out with a short small bore needle. Complete kits are available – Leader-Cath. A guide wire with a J shaped tip increases successful catheterisation of the external jugular vein – Hydrocath.

A stylet is useful to thread the catheter forward and to indicate the length of catheter in the patient. The presumptive position of the tip can be estimated and the catheter withdrawn if necessary so that the tip lies above the nipple line. A precoiled catheter (inside a drum) can be more frequently placed in the superior vena cava.

The table provides guidance on choosing the appropriate sized equipment.

Methods

Sites of entry to central venous system

Arm veins
External jugular vein
Internal jugular vein
Infraclavicular subclavian vein

The techniques are described in order of safety and effectiveness. In each, air embolism is avoided by maintaining the venous pressure above atmospheric by position or a tourniquet on the limb. If the patient is conscious the skin should be infiltrated with a local anaesthetic using a fine needle.

Arm veins

The median (basilic) arm veins are the safest approach to the central venous system. The cephalic vein curves sharply to join the axillary vein through the deep fascia at the shoulder, which may impede passage of a catheter. This results in less successful central placement, but it is still worth attempting. The veins are distended by a tourniquet. The head is turned to the same side to compress the neck veins, and the arm is abducted. The catheter should be of 600 mm minimum length. When the tourniquet is released air embolism may occur, so depress the proximal end of the catheter below the level of the patient's elbow.

External jugular vein

The external jugular vein runs from the angle of the mandible to behind the middle of the clavicle and joins the subclavian vein. The patient is placed on a 20° head down position with the head turned to the opposite side. The most prominent vein is chosen. If neither vein becomes visible or palpable cannulation is inadvisable. In about half the attempts the catheter cannot be threaded into an intrathoracic vein, but successful central placement may be helped by digital pressure above the clavicle, by depressing the shoulder, or by flushing saline through the catheter. The use of a Seldinger wire or a spiral J shaped wire increases the incidence of successful central placement of the catheter and its use is strongly recommended. The use of excessive force should be avoided. Satisfactory measurement of central venous pressure is sometimes possible from the external jugular vein or from the junction of the external jugular and subclavian veins. This junction is a common site for the distal tip to lodge when the catheter will not thread centrally.

Internal jugular vein

The internal jugular veins run behind the sternomastoid close to the lateral border of the carotid artery. One easy way of finding the vein is to rest the pads of the fingers on the side of the larynx with the tips of the fingers pointing backwards. The carotid artery is then behind the finger tips and the internal jugular vein lies just lateral to the artery. It is advisable to enter the vein at, or above, the level of the cricoid cartilage, to minimise the risk of damaging structures in the root of the neck (Fig 3a). It is helpful to draw a line across the neck with a marker pen. The line is drawn just above the level of the cricoid cartilage and helps in identifying the skin entry point.

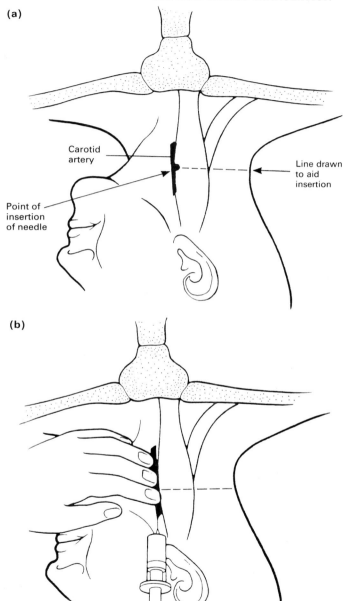

(a)

Carotid artery

Line drawn to aid insertion

Point of insertion of needle

(b)

FIG 3

(c) Elevate syringe 45° above skin surface

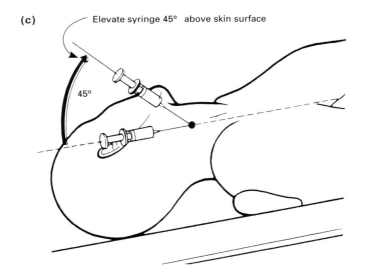

45°

FIG 3   Internal jugular vein puncture. (Reproduced, with permission, from M Rosen, IP Latto and WS Ng. *Handbook of Percutaneous Central Venous Catheterisation*, 2nd edn. London: WB Saunders, 1992)

The patient is placed in a 20° head down position with the head turned to the left. The neck should be slightly extended and all pillows removed. Cannulation of the right vein is preferred to avoid injury to the thoracic duct and because it is technically easier for a right handed operator. If a Seldinger wire technique is used the operator should wear gown and gloves. The needle is inserted just lateral to the fingers of the left hand (with the fingertips pointing backwards over the carotid artery) (Fig 3b). The needle is directed towards the feet, parallel to the midline with the syringe raised 30–45° above the skin (Fig 3c). Gentle aspiration is maintained as the needle is advanced. A flush of blood into the syringe confirms entry of blood into the vein. It is recommended that these steps should be carried out first, using a small (21 gauge) needle to locate the vein, before proceeding with the larger needle. This minimises trauma caused by the large needle if the vein is hard to find. If the vein is not located at the first pass with the seeker needle then the needle should be slowly withdrawn and redirected in a more lateral direction. There should be a limit (five) to the number of attempts at entering the vein with the large needle. Remove the large needle if the carotid artery is accidentally punctured and apply firm pressure to the neck for five minutes. This minimises the risk of a haematoma.

Infraclavicular subclavian vein

The subclavian vein is particularly suitable for administering long term parenteral nutrition. Infraclavicular subclavian vein catheters are more comfortable for the patient, do not restrict neck and arm movements, and facilitate nursing care of the catheter. It is widely patent even in states of circulatory collapse, so that subclavian venepuncture may provide the only route for rapid infusion. Puncture and catheterisation of the subclavian vein is a blind procedure. Serious harm can be inflicted on nearby vital structures and deaths have been reported. The most common complication is pneumothorax. The procedure, therefore, should not ordinarily be performed by an inexperienced operator without close supervision. The subclavian vein lies in the angle formed by the medial one third of the clavicle and the first rib, in which the subclavian vein crosses over the first rib to enter the thoracic cavity. There is some variation in the anatomy of this region, which has prompted the use of an ultrasonic probe to facilitate locating the position of the subclavian vein. This manoeuvre, however, is unlikely to reduce the incidence of pneumothorax.

The patient rests supine, tilted 20° head down. Either side may be used, although the right side is preferable. The patient's head is turned to the opposite side. The following landmarks (Fig 4a) are identified: the midpoint of the clavicle; the triangle formed by the sternal and clavicular heads of the sternomastoid muscle; and the suprasternal notch. A guide wire technique is recommended. The needle is attached to a saline filled syringe and is inserted below the midpoint of the clavicle. The needle is pointed at the small triangle formed by the heads of the sternomastoid muscle and the clavicle (Fig 4a). Alternatively, if this triangle is not easily defined, the needle is directed towards the suprasternal notch, keeping a finger tip in the notch to act as a target (Fig 4b). The needle tip is advanced slowly close to the undersurface of the clavicle, keeping needle and syringe parallel to the coronal plane (Fig 4c). While the needle is advanced gentle aspiration should be maintained, and a

(a)

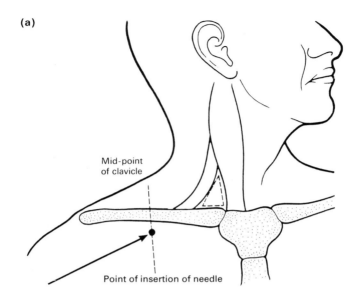

Mid-point
of clavicle

Point of insertion of needle

(b)

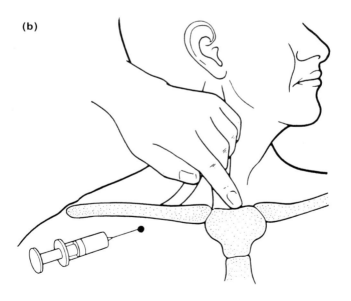

(c)

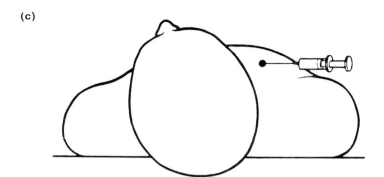

FIG 4   Infraclavicular subclavian vein puncture. (Reproduced, with permission, from M Rosen, IP Latto and WS Ng. *Handbook of Percutaneous Central Venous Catheterisation*, 2nd edn. London: WB Saunders, 1992)

flush of blood indicates that the vein is entered. If the attempt is unsuccessful, further attempts may be made, altering the direction of the needle only when it has been withdrawn to just beneath the skin. A chest radiograph should always be taken to check for pneumothorax.

Checking and testing

Blood should be aspirated freely to ensure that the catheter is in a vascular space before injecting fluid. If the line is connected to a bottle of fluid that is lowered below the patient, blood should flow freely under the influence of gravity. On connection to a column of fluid for measurements of central venous pressure the fluid column should show slow oscillations related to respiration and quicker oscillations related to the heart beats. A chest radiograph (Fig 5) should be taken to confirm that the position of the tip is above the right atrium, preferably not more than 2 cm below a line joining the lower borders of the clavicles.

Management

Fixing the catheter (Fig 6)

Once satisfactorily placed, the catheter should be fixed carefully to prevent inadvertent withdrawal or movement further into the

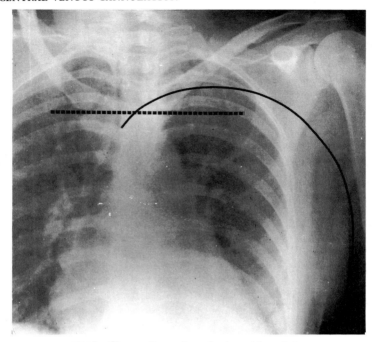

FIG 5   Chest radiograph to check position of tip

vein. Firm fixation probably also reduces the incidence of thrombophlebitis. Adhesive tape (1 cm wide) is crossed over to grip the
catheter firmly, away from the venepuncture site. An alternative,
especially for longer term use, is to secure the catheter with a skin
suture.

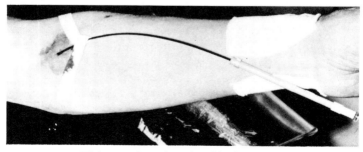

FIG 6   Fixing a catheter introduced in the antecubital fossa

The puncture site is sprayed with an antiseptic preparation such as povidone–iodine, then a plastic wound dressing, and finally covered with a transparent, occlusive dressing.

Asepsis

The most scrupulous attention to detail is needed to keep venous catheters infection free. Strict aseptic technique during the insertion of the catheter is essential. Additions to intravenous fluids should preferably be introduced in the aseptic laboratory of the pharmacy. The intravenous giving set should be changed daily, an aseptic technique being used while connecting it to the catheter. Injecting drugs into the venous catheter and taking blood samples through stopcocks should be avoided if possible. Injections should be made through latex covered ports which can be swabbed with antiseptic before insertion of a needle. Regular bacteriological monitoring of the venepuncture site should be carried out. It is important to be vigilant to detect catheter related infections. If an infection occurs the catheter may have to be removed.

Clotting

A continuous flow through the catheter prevents reflux of blood and clotting. When the catheter is not in immediate use, it should be filled with heparinised saline.

Complications

Complications of central venous catheterisation mostly fall into two categories – first, those that occur at the time of catheterisation and result from injury to some vital structure; and, second, those that occur at a later stage and are associated with catheter related thrombophlebitis and infection. In addition to these two groups air embolism, catheter embolism, cardiac arrhythmias, and perforation of the myocardium may occur at any time. Suspicion should be aroused if there are unexplained cardiovascular disturbances. Perforation into the mediastinum or pericardium may be recognised only on a routine chest radiograph. An offending catheter should be withdrawn to a safer position and any infusion stopped. Timely application of a tourniquet may prevent a sheared off catheter migrating up an arm vein. A catheter embolus requires early intervention for its removal. Disturbances of cardiac rhythm

Complications

Immediate	Immediate or later	Later
Arterial puncture	Air embolism	Myocardial
Cardiac arrhythmias	Catheter embolus	perforation and
Injury to thoracic	Pneumothorax	tamponade
duct		Hydrothorax
Injury to nerves		Infection
		Venous thrombosis

stimulated by a catheter in the heart usually subside spontaneously but, if not, the catheter should be withdrawn into the superior vena cava. Persistent severe arrhythmias require urgent treatment. When arm or external jugular veins are used serious immediate complications are rare. The veins are usually visible and palpable. Catheters lying in peripheral veins, however, often lead to thrombophlebitis if left in position for more than one or two days. Most immediate and serious complications are a feature of blind venepuncture of the subclavian and, to a lesser extent, internal jugular veins. Injury to many structures related to the thoracic inlet has been reported: pneumothorax, haemothorax, arterial puncture, and damage to the thoracic duct and phrenic nerve. The need for insertion of a chest drain will depend on the size of the pneumothorax and the respiratory embarrassment it causes. Drainage is required if the pneumothorax is 50% or more. If smaller, observation of the patient and a repeat chest radiograph in 4–6 hours (more frequently in patients on positive pressure ventilation) will reveal an increasing pneumothorax. A tension pneumothorax requires immediate drainage with a small bore needle. A haematoma in the neck associated with arterial puncture is usually controlled by applying firm pressure for five minutes. Close observation of the site should be continued. Surgical repair is only rarely needed. The complication rates reported after catheterisation of the deep veins range between 0 and 15% and are probably dependent on the experience of the operator.

7 Temporary cardiac pacing

S BURN
PC BARNES

Temporary transvenous pacing is a procedure that any doctor concerned with acute coronary care may be called on to perform. This procedure is often carried out by junior staff when emergency heart rate support is required for the patient's survival. Both the skill of central vein cannulation and a sound knowledge of the indications for, and contraindications to, temporary pacing are required.

The vast majority of temporary pacing wires are used for right ventricular endocardial pacing, which is described here.

Indications (Box A)

The indications for temporary pacing can be divided into five main groups:

- Myocardial infarction
- Non-cardiac surgery with a risk of bradycardia
- Symptomatic bradycardia in other situations
- Overdrive suppression of tachycardias
- Managing an asystolic cardiac arrest.

Contraindications

These include:

- Prosthetic tricuspid valve
- Tricuspid stenosis.

Box A

Myocardial infarction

Anterior myocardial infarction
Complete atrioventricular block
Mobitz type II second degree block
Alternating right and left bundle branch block
Right bundle branch block and new left posterior hemiblock
Right bundle branch block and left anterior hemiblock, and first degree atrioventricular block
Left bundle branch block and first degree atrioventricular block
Symptomatic bradycardia resistant to atropine

Inferior myocardial infarction
Any of the above associated with haemodynamic compromise and resistant to atropine, except complete heart block
Complete atrioventricular block if ventricular rate under 40/min or associated with heart failure, low output state, or ventricular arrhythmias

Cover for general anaesthesia
Complete atrioventricular block
Second degree atrioventricular block (Mobitz II)
Bifascicular block and first degree heart block
 ie, right bundle branch block, left posterior hemiblock, and primary heart block
 right bundle branch block, left anterior hemiblock, and primary heart block
 left bundle branch block and primary heart block
Intermittent atrioventricular block
Second degree atrioventricular block (Mobitz I), left bundle branch block, or bifascicular block *only* if associated with a history of syncope

Symptomatic bradycardia
Symptoms associated with bradycardias caused by high degree atrioventricular block or sinoatrial disease when permanent pacing is not immediately available
As a cover for cardioversion of a tachycardia associated with the "tachycardia–bradycardia syndrome" (profound bradycardia can occur post-cardioversion)
Some drug overdoses, eg, β blocker

Overdrive suppression

Occasionally required for the overdrive pacing of ventricular or atrial arrhythmias resistant to drug therapy

Cardiac arrest

Emergency pacing may be indicated in some asystolic arrests *if* evidence of electrical activity – particularly independent "p" wave activity. Try transcutaneous pacing as a holding measure while preparing for transvenous pacing

Thrombolysis and pacing

In a coronary care unit a problem that is not uncommon is the patient who requires a temporary pacemaker and who also requires, or more usually has already received, thrombolytic therapy. Central venous cannulation in such patients has inherent risks, particularly if the arterial circulation is inadvertently entered. Non-invasive transcutaneous pacing can be used as a holding measure. If, however, transvenous pacing is definitely indicated then the insertion site must be carefully chosen. The subclavian vein should be avoided because it, and the subclavian artery, are impossible to compress adequately in the event of bleeding.

The preferred sites of entry, in these patients, are the right internal jugular vein and the right femoral vein. The femoral vein is probably the safest, provided the femoral artery is easily palpable. It also has the advantage of providing an approach to the right atrium from below, and often placement of the wire in the apex of the right ventricle is relatively easy. The femoral route should only be used for short periods – usually 48 hours or less.

Transcutaneous pacing

Non-invasive transcutaneous pacing equipment is becoming more widely available now and the technique is useful in patients with contraindications to transvenous pacing, or where there will be a delay in instituting it. The procedure uses an external signal generator (often attached to a defibrillator system) which stimulates the heart via external pads placed on the chest wall. It is well tolerated by patients for some hours until alternative methods are sought.

79

Equipment

Equipment

Chlorhexidine or iodine skin preparation
Sterile towels
Sterile gown and gloves
Lignocaine 1% local anaesthetic, needles, and syringes
A small blade
Suture material
Introducer needle for central vein with guide wire and sheath
Bipolar ventricular pacing wire
Connector cable to generator
Pulse generator box
Radiographic screening facility

Pacing wires

These wires are usually 5 or 6 French gauge plastic disposable bipolar wires. Many come with their own introducer needles and cannulas, although the use of a separate introducer sheath is preferable. They are usually inserted using the Seldinger guide wire technique and have separate side-ports for drug administration if required. Many such sheaths have small rubber haemostatic valves which allow replacement of pacing wires without having to remove the sheath itself.

Pulse generator

Two major types of generator box are usually available, with the smaller being suitable for ambulant patients (Fig 1).

Controls on the boxes are used to set the pacing rate and the output voltage. Needles or lights on the generator indicate when it is sensing or pacing. Most generator boxes can be set for fixed rate or demand pacing, although in almost all cases demand pacing is the desired mode.

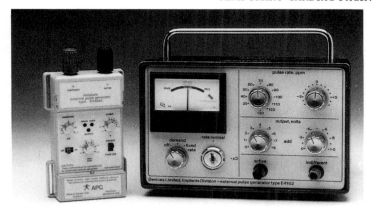

FIG 1   The two different sizes of pulse generator box

Procedure

Precautions
- Ensure a defibrillator and facilities for emergency trancutaneous pacing are available
- The procedure is performed under radiographic screening using fluoroscopy
- Antibiotic cover should be considered for patients with known or suspected valvular or congenital heart disease
- Patients receiving thrombolytic therapy (see above)
- Consider monitoring oxygen saturation during the procedure (using pulse oximetry), particularly in "sick" patients

Sites of insertion

In patients not receiving thrombolytic therapy, the infra-clavicular approach to the right subclavian vein is the preferred route. It offers a stable position which is relatively easy to keep sterile and does not hinder the patient's mobility. It also leaves the left subclavian vessels available for permanent pacing, if required.

Alternative routes include the internal jugular, femoral, or antecubital veins.

81

Cannulation

The chosen vein is cannulated under full asepsis with the patient supine. The Seldinger technique of catheter-over-guide wire is the preferred method.

The technique of central vein cannulation is described in Chapter 6. Once the vein is entered, a guide wire is inserted through the needle and directed towards the right atrium. If in doubt, the position of the guide wire should be checked via fluoroscopy before a dilator and sheath are passed over it.

Once the sheath is inserted and has been flushed with saline, the pacing wire can be passed through it, ready for positioning in the right ventricle under radiographic control.

Positioning

This is shown in Figure 2a–e.

Threshold

Once positioned in the right ventricular apex, connect the pacing wire to the pulse generator via the connecting lead (positive and negative contacts). The pulse duration is usually 2 ms and is internally set by the generator.

Set the output voltage at 3 V and the rate at 70 beats/min or 10 beats/min faster than the patient's own rate. The generator should be in the demand pacing mode.

Successful pacing capture will show pacing spikes on the monitor with ventricular complexes (Fig 3).

Reduce the output voltage gradually until pacing capture is just lost – this is the pacing threshold. To be acceptable it should be $\leqslant 1$ V. If it is not and the patient's state allows, reposition the wire after turning off the generator and disconnecting.

Check the stability of the final position by ensuring that there is continued pacing during deep inspiration and coughing.

Set the output voltage to two or three times the measured threshold. The threshold itself should be checked daily and the output voltage adjusted accordingly. The pacing threshold commonly rises to two or three times the initial value during the first few days.

Leave the generator in "demand" mode at an appropriate rate; if in sinus rhythm set at 50 beats/min as "back-up"; if in heart block set at 70–80 beats/min to start with.

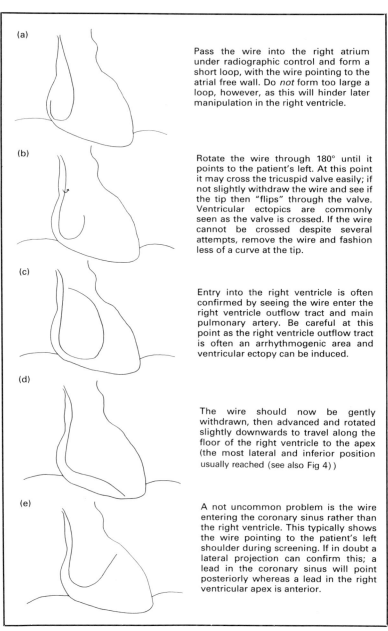

(a) Pass the wire into the right atrium under radiographic control and form a short loop, with the wire pointing to the atrial free wall. Do *not* form too large a loop, however, as this will hinder later manipulation in the right ventricle.

(b) Rotate the wire through 180° until it points to the patient's left. At this point it may cross the tricuspid valve easily; if not slightly withdraw the wire and see if the tip then "flips" through the valve. Ventricular ectopics are commonly seen as the valve is crossed. If the wire cannot be crossed despite several attempts, remove the wire and fashion less of a curve at the tip.

(c) Entry into the right ventricle is often confirmed by seeing the wire enter the right ventricle outflow tract and main pulmonary artery. Be careful at this point as the right ventricle outflow tract is often an arrhythmogenic area and ventricular ectopy can be induced.

(d) The wire should now be gently withdrawn, then advanced and rotated slightly downwards to travel along the floor of the right ventricle to the apex (the most lateral and inferior position usually reached (see also Fig 4))

(e) A not uncommon problem is the wire entering the coronary sinus rather than the right ventricle. This typically shows the wire pointing to the patient's left shoulder during screening. If in doubt a lateral projection can confirm this; a lead in the coronary sinus will point posteriorly whereas a lead in the right ventricular apex is anterior.

FIG 2 Positioning of pacing wire

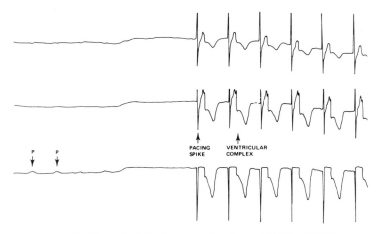

FIG 3 Three-lead rhythm strip showing ventricular capture

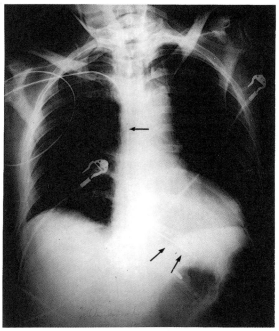

FIG 4 Chest radiograph taken on a portable machine, showing a temporary wire in situ (see also Fig 2d)

Aftercare

- Once the position is accepted, screen the wire to ensure that there are no redundant loops in the right atrium
- Suture the electrode at the point of exit from the skin with 2/0 silk but take care not to damage the insulation. Cover with a dressing. The rest of the wire can be looped and fixed to the skin with tape
- Obtain a chest radiograph to confirm the position of the wire and exclude a pneumothorax. An ideal position is shown in Fig 4

Pacing

Problems

1	No pacing spikes seen:	Can be caused by pulse generator failure or loose connection, or "oversensing" of patient's own electrical activity causing inhibition of the generator
2	Pacing spikes seen but no ventricular capture:	Can be caused by electrode displacement, myocardial perforation, or increasing threshold ("exit block")
3	Pericardial pain:	Occasionally seen even in the absence of perforation. Ensure threshold stable and check for signs of perforation (see below)
4	Myocardial perforation:	Patient usually develops chest pain with loss of pacing capture. Can see pacing of the diaphragm. Cardiac tamponade is rare and usually the wire merely needs repositioning or replacing
5	Diaphragmatic pacing:	Usually indicates perforation but can be seen if the output voltage is set too high

Duration

In the case of symptomatic chronic atrioventricular nodal or sinoatrial disease, temporary pacing will be stopped once permanent pacing has been started.

With acute myocardial infarction, normal atrioventricular conduction often returns after a few days. However, this can be delayed for up to three weeks.

Patients with anterior infarction often have evidence of persistent bundle branch damage. The question of permanent pacemakers in this group is still controversial and should be discussed with a cardiologist if a permanent system is thought to be indicated.

Wires inserted via the femoral vein should be removed within 48 h if possible because of the risks of infection and/or venous thrombosis.

8 Chest drains

J AU
T HOOPER

Insertion of a chest drain is one of the more invasive procedures that the newly qualified houseman or inexperienced senior house officer may be called on to perform, sometimes in a life-threatening emergency. With surface anatomy a distant memory and the spectre of injury to major organs an ever present danger, it is not surprising that this procedure has engendered a disproportionate amount of anxiety and even fear in generations of ill-prepared juniors. However, provided a few simple rules are followed, chest drain insertion can be achieved with the minimum amount of angst and a high degree of safety.

Indications

Intercostal intubation is indicated for the drainage of air, fluid, or pus *that can be aspirated via an exploratory 18 gauge needle.*

Indications for chest drainage

- Air
    Spontaneous
    Traumatic
    Iatrogenic
    Bronchopleural fistula
- Fluid
    Haemothorax
    Chylothorax
    Malignant effusion
    Benign effusion
- Pus
    Empyema
    Parapneumonic effusion

Contraindications

Intercostal intubation is contraindicated when *exploratory needle aspiration is negative*, a bleeding diathesis exists, or the operator is inexperienced and has no supervision.

Equipment

Most wards or casualty departments will have pre-packed and sterilised intercostal intubation sets (Fig 1). Note that a chest drain is not included in the intubation set because it is impractical to include tubes of a whole range of sizes. The other items that you must ensure are present before you start are shown in the box.

- Sterile syringes (5 and 10 ml)
- Local anaesthetic (10 ml 1% plain lignocaine)
- Skin antiseptic solution
- No. 11 scalpel blade
- "0" or "1" silk or nylon drain stitch
- Sterile gloves
- Sterile gown
- Underwater seal drainage bottle and tubing
- Dressings

Surface anatomy and insertion sites

For the emergency relief of tension pneumothorax, the chest drain is usually inserted anteriorly in the second intercostal space (Fig 2). However, the preferred site of entry for chest drainage is the fourth or fifth intercostal space laterally (Fig 3), because it is associated with the least discomfort, allows for better mobility, and is cosmetically superior, especially in women. More posteriorly placed drains are not recommended: they are very uncomfortable and the tubes become kinked as the patient lies back. Likewise, drains inserted below nipple level are to be deplored: there is an ever present risk of injury to intra-abdominal organs.

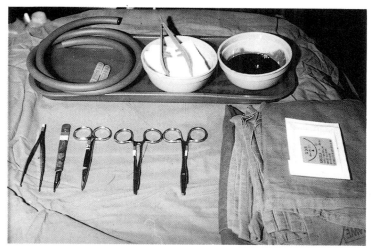

FIG 1   Contents of typical chest drain pack (clockwise from top left): (1) drain tubing, (2) bowl and gauze swabs, (3) skin antiseptic solution, (4) drapes, (5) Spencer–Wells artery forceps, (6) scissors, (7) scalpel handle and blade, and (8) tissue forceps. Many packs contain Tudor–Edwards trocars and cannulas: medium (8 mm or 22 French gauge) and large (9·5 mm or 28 French gauge), for the insertion of drains without trocars

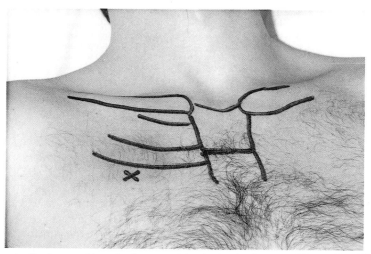

FIG 2   Surface markings for intercostal intubation in the second interspace. The chest drain is inserted in the mid-clavicular line. The patient lies semi-reclined at 30° with the head turned away from the operative site

89

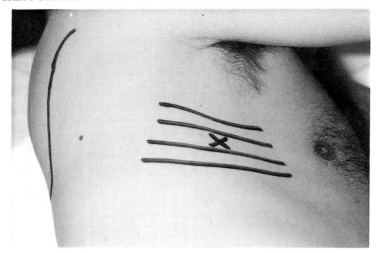

FIG 3 Surface markings for intercostal intubation in the fourth or fifth interspace. The chest drain is inserted in the mid-axillary line just behind the lateral border of the pectoral muscles, at about nipple level. The patient lies on his or her side with the arm extended

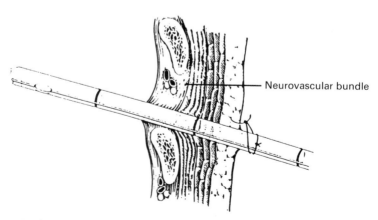

FIG 4 Anatomy of intercostal space showing ideal route for drain insertion

On full expiration, the right dome of the diaphragm is level with the fourth interspace or right nipple, and the left dome of the diaphragm with the fifth rib or 0·5 inch (13 mm) below the left nipple

Procedure

Before performing the procedure, explain to the patient what you are going to do and why. During the procedure, tell the patient what you are doing step by step: this will go a long way towards allaying your patient's anxiety. Even in the most experienced hands, effective local anaesthesia can sometimes be difficult to achieve. Administration of a small dose of midazolam (2–3 mg) can often provide complete amnesia for the procedure, assuming no contraindications to intravenous sedation exist.

- **Inspect** the chest radiograph and locate the surface markings for intubation
- **Explore** with an 18 gauge needle
- **Create** a track
- **Insert** the chest drain

We cannot over-emphasise the importance of obtaining a positive tap before proceeding to chest intubation. Blind intubations are not recommended even in experienced hands: the rate of failed intubation and the risk of damage to intrathoracic organs are unacceptably high. The exploratory tap and local anaesthesia can usefully be combined in the one manoeuvre: with local anaesthetic in a 10 ml syringe attached to an 18 gauge needle, the skin over the selected rib space is first anaesthetised. The needle is then advanced until contact is made with the rib below the space selected, "walked" over the *top* of the rib, and advanced into the pleural cavity, while continually withdrawing on the syringe. The appearance of air or fluid indicates a successful tap.

The neurovascular bundle lies immediately below the rib of the corresponding space in the costal groove (Fig 4)

While still withdrawing on the syringe, the needle is withdrawn until it lies just outside the pleural cavity. A liberal amount of local anaesthetic is injected widely in this plane to anaesthetise the sensitive parietal pleura and the intercostal nerve above. Following this, the periosteum of the rib below is infiltrated. If pus is aspirated, the contaminated syringe is replaced with a fresh one before infiltration of local anaesthetic.

Chest intubation (Figs 5–7)

Full aseptic precautions must be applied. The procedure is shown in the box.

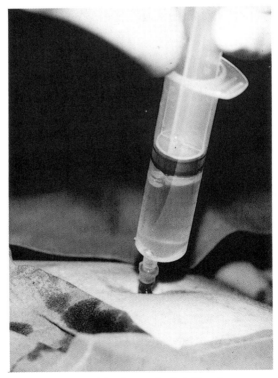

FIG 5   Exploratory aspiration and local anaesthetic infiltration

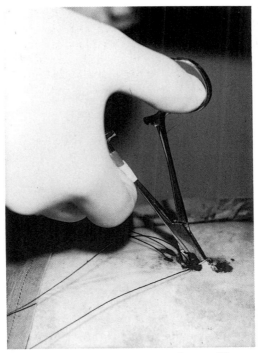

FIG 6   Creation of drain track with blunt artery forceps. The trocar chest drain is then inserted without force. Just inside the pleural cavity, the trocar is withdrawn and the drain directed to the appropriate site

- Skin incision
- Insert purse-string and drain stitch
- Create track with blunt artery forceps
- Measure length of drain to insert
- Insert chest drain without undue force
- Clamp and secure drain in place
- Connect to underwater seal and unclamp
- Check for bubbling or drainage of fluid, and respiratory swing
- Repeat radiograph

The most important step in the whole procedure is the creation of a track with blunt artery forceps. With gentle but firm pressure, the forceps are advanced over the upper border of the selected rib into the intercostal space. A controlled increase in force while

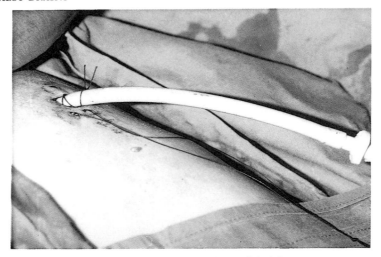

FIG 7   Chest drain secured in place and draining pus

gently opening and closing the jaws of the forceps will be rewarded by a "pop" as it penetrates the parietal pleura. This is usually accompanied by the escape of air or fluid. The jaws of the forceps are then opened widely in two planes to create a track, which should be large enough to allow introduction of the chest drain with minimal force. The trocar drain or trocar cannula can now be inserted with ease, without fear of injury to intrathoracic organs. For drainage of air, the drain should be directed towards the apex of the chest. For drainage of fluid, the drain should be directed towards the base.

The easiest part of the procedure to forget is measurement of the length of tube for insertion. Too long an insertion may result in kinking and a non-functioning tube; too short an insertion may result in embarrassing subcutaneous placement.

94

Size of tube

A large tube (28–32 French gauge) is necessary for the drainage of blood or pus, whereas smaller tubes are sufficient for the drainage of air or serous effusions. Tubes as small as 8 French gauge have been used successfully for the drainage of serous effusions, but are not recommended for drainage that is expected to last for more than 24 hours. Small tubes kink easily and become obstructed by intraluminal deposits of fibrin and debris, often necessitating further tube placement. For practical purposes, the smallest tube that we would recommend is 20 French gauge.

Tube management

Suction applied to the underwater seal at 0·98–1·96 kPa (10–20 cm H_2O) increases the efficiency of the drainage system. Only a high volume, low pressure pump should be used (eg, a Vernon–Thompson pump). Wall suction units can also be used provided an adaptor is employed to reduce the pressure. Complete drainage of pleural collections and re-expansion of the lung should be confirmed by serial chest radiographs. Patients with a subacute or chronic empyema should be referred for thoracic surgical management. Drains should not be clamped for prolonged periods during patient transportation, and should *never* be clamped if still bubbling, because tension may result.

Tube removal

Chest drains can be removed 24 hours after drainage of air or fluid has ceased. Check for air leaks by asking the patient to cough and noting the escape of bubbles. At the time of removal, the patient should inhale fully and perform a Valsalva manoeuvre. The chest drain is removed sharply and the purse-string suture tied. During removal of the drain it is quite acceptable to keep the drain on suction. A check radiograph is traditionally advised immediately following drain removal, but is probably unnecessary provided the correct technique has been applied and the patient is clinically well. A chest radiograph should, however, be done 24 hours later to check for re-accumulation of air or fluid.

95

Complications

Complications of intercostal drainage
- Incorrect placement
- Visceral injury
    lung
    heart
    diaphragm
    liver
    spleen
    stomach
- Injury to intercostal artery
- Re-expansion pulmonary oedema
- Empyema

Incorrectly placed tubes should be re-sited. Accidental penetration of viscera should be promptly referred to a thoracic or general surgical unit for further management. Injury to intercostal vessels may necessitate thoracotomy and is avoided by passing the drain close to the upper border of the rib (see Fig 4). Re-expansion pulmonary oedema is a rare complication of rapid drainage of a large effusion, and can be avoided by limiting the initial drainage to 1 l/hour. Prolonged drainage (> 10 days) increases the risk of intrapleural infection; however, there is no convincing evidence that prophylactic antibiotics are beneficial.

9 Pericardial aspiration

AA GEHANI

Indications

1 As an emergency procedure to relieve cardiac tamponade
2 To obtain samples of pericardial fluid for analysis – for example, culture, cytology

Pericardial puncture should *not* be undertaken to ascertain whether a pericardial effusion is present. Before embarking on the procedure, carefully consider the evidence that an effusion (or haemopericardium) exists.

Diagnosis

Clinical signs

The clinical presentation is a result of speed of accumulation and volume of pericardial effusion. Small but rapid collection causes profound haemodynamic effects whereas large chronic effusions can be well tolerated. The physical signs of tamponade may be difficult to interpret, the chief alternative diagnosis obviously being cardiac failure from any cause. The picture of acute or progressive cardiac tamponade is one of circulatory embarrassment with tachycardia, raised jugular venous pressure, small pulse pressure, hypotension, muffled heart sounds, and pulsus paradoxus.

97

Pulsus paradoxus is elicited by allowing a very slow fall in sphygmomanometer cuff pressure while the subject breathes regularly and a little more deeply than normal. Occasionally the sign may be detectable on palpation of major pulses. The magnitude of the "paradoxus" is the difference in systolic blood pressure between the first hearing of the Korotkoff sounds on expiration only and the point at which they become continuous in both phases of respiration. (The term "paradoxus" is strictly a misnomer, because the phasic difference is simply an exaggeration of the inspiratory fall in systolic pressure seen in normal subjects, but is not usually readily detected.)

Remember that a pericardial rub is unlikely to be present with a sizeable effusion and that cardiac tamponade constituting an emergency cannot be present without raised jugular venous pressure.

Echocardiography (Figs 1–3)

Echocardiography is the single most reliable and practical method of proving a pericardial effusion and of assessing its volume or demonstrating loculation. Signs of cardiac embarrassment on M-mode tracing and two-dimensional pictures require skilled interpretation. The ultrasonic beam will show a space between the pericardium and the anterior right and/or posterior left ventricular wall.

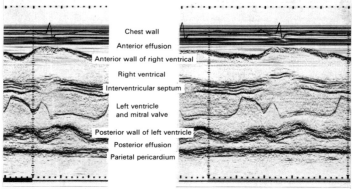

Chest wall
Anterior effusion
Anterior wall of right ventrical
Right ventrical
Interventricular septum
Left ventricle and mitral valve
Posterior wall of left ventricle
Posterior effusion
Parietal pericardium

FIG 1   M-mode echocardiogram revealing an echo "free" space anteriorly and posteriorly which indicates accumulation of pericardial fluid. Note the "paradoxical" movement of the septum

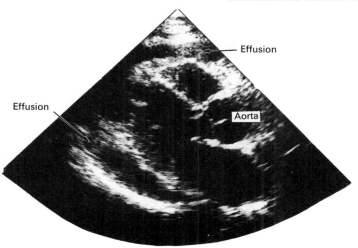

FIG 2   Two-dimensional echocardiogram of a patient with large pericardial effusion

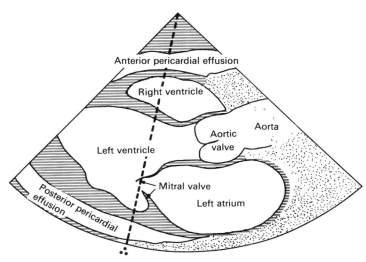

Triangular plane of corresponding M mode

FIG 3   Diagram highlighting the structures seen in Fig 2. The cursor corresponds to the M-mode seen in Fig 1

99

Chest radiography (Figs 4 and 5)

Cardiac size on chest radiograph is a function of the volume and chronicity of pericardial effusion. When time has allowed stretching of the pericardium, the cardiac silhouette may be grossly enlarged and appear pear shaped, with bulging over the right atrium and apex. Gross enlargement is often seen in slowly accumulating effusion, but remember that a life-threatening acute tamponade (for example, haemorrhage from trauma) can be present with little or no cardiac enlargement on the chest radiograph.

Electrocardiography

The ECG does not provide reliable evidence of pericardial

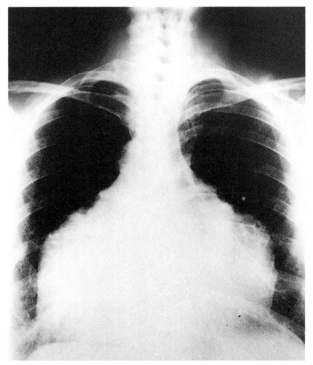

FIG 4   Chest radiograph showing typical appearance of a large pericardial effusion

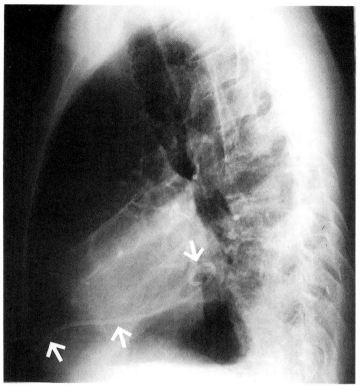

FIG 5 Lateral chest radiograph demonstrating the course of a "pigtail" catheter into the pericardium with the tip in the posterior pericardium (white arrows)

tamponade or effusion. The presence of low, voltage complexes should not be regarded as a specific diagnostic sign.

Contraindications

The main contraindication is doubt about whether an effusion is present. After cardiac surgery (or possibly radiotherapy), loculation of fluid and adhesions may increase the hazard of the procedure.

101

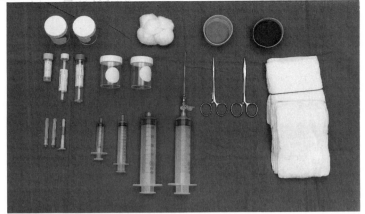

FIG 6 Display of the basic instruments required for pericardiocentesis

Equipment (Fig 6)

- Sterilisation fluid for skin (iodine, chlorhexidine)
- Sterile drapes
- Syringes and needles for injection of local anaesthetic (1–2% lignocaine)
- 18 gauge lumbar puncture needle
- Three way tap
- 50 ml aspiration syringe(s)
- Spencer–Wells forceps
- Specimen containers
- Standby resuscitation trolley (DC defibrillator, intravenous atropine, saline, etc)
- J-tipped floppy guide wire
- Dilator and short pigtail catheter (5 French gauge size)

Before you start

Explain the procedure to the patient, who should be undressed to the waist and reclining comfortably in bed with the thorax at an angle of 30–45° to the horizontal. He or she should be connected to an electrocardiography (ECG) monitor, and an intravenous line or cannula should be inserted and kept open by slow saline drip. If he or she is tense or anxious an intravenous injection of diazepam (perhaps 5–10 mg) may make the procedure easier for both the

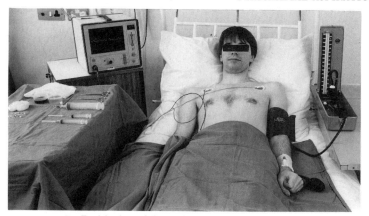

FIG 7   Positioning of the patient and accessory attachments

patient and the operator. The operator should wear mask, gown, and gloves. The skin at the puncture site should be well cleaned and a sterile towel placed over the abdomen and legs. Blood pressure should be documented immediately before the procedure and the cuff left in place.

Procedure

Xiphisternal route

The safest and the recommended route is through the angle between the xiphoid process and the left costal margin. This approach is extrapleural aiming at traversing the membranous portion of the diaphragm. The skin and deep tissues are infiltrated with 10 ml 2% lignocaine solution. The puncture needle is attached to a 10 ml syringe containing 3 ml 2% lignocaine. This is to clear the needle and provide anaesthesia to deep structures. The needle is aimed posteriorly at an angle of 30–40° to the skin in the approximate direction of the left shoulder. The object is to traverse the diaphragm opposite the middle of the diaphragmatic surface of the heart. The needle is advanced slowly, with gentle suction, until the pericardial sac is entered and fluid aspirated. Insertion of the needle some 5–7 cm (2–2·5 inches) will usually be required before the pericardium is reached.

The ECG monitor should be watched during insertion of the

103

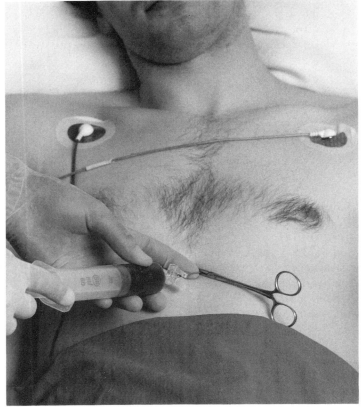

FIG 8   Aspiration of a "bloody" pericardial effusion via the subxiphoid route. Note the direction of the needle. The Spencer–Wells forceps prevents inadvertent advance of the needle

needle for occurrence of ectopic beats or any other changes. If the needle is advanced too far the myocardium will be felt knocking against the tip or will cause the needle to waggle. If this occurs withdraw the needle; never advance it further.

A Spencer–Wells forceps is clamped to the needle next to the skin to prevent further inadvertent penetration. By using the syringe and three way tap, fluid is aspirated, and samples are sent for culture, cytology, and so on.

104

A blood stained effusion may be distinguished from blood aspirated from the heart by placing a sample in a glass specimen bottle. The effusion will not clot, the aspirate will (except in cases of coagulopathy).

Placement of an intrapericardial catheter

Needle aspiration is often all that is required to relieve acute tamponade; however, if rapid reaccumulation is anticipated or if administration of intrapericardial drugs is required, an "atraumatic" catheter should replace the needle using a modified Seldinger technique. This should be carried out while there is still some fluid in the pericardium as follows.

Introduce a floppy J-tipped guide wire through the needle which is then replaced by a dilator. Remove the dilator and slide a short pigtail or similar "soft" catheter over the wire. Remove the wire and attach a three way stopcock. Secure to the skin by silk suture or plaster (see Fig 5).

A decision to place an intrapericardial catheter should be made before starting the procedure and the required equipment should be ready. *Do not* leave the sharp needle in the pericardium while calling for additional instruments.

Apical route

The needle is introduced at the cardiac apex in the fourth or fifth intercostal space 2 cm medial to the lateral edge of the cardiac dullness. This route carries a greater risk of injury to the pleura and the coronary arteries, as well as contamination of the pleural space when the pericardial fluid is purulent.

Parasternal route

The needle is introduced in the fifth left intercostal space just to the left of the sternum and aimed straight backwards. The internal mammary artery lies 2 cm lateral to the sternal edge and the needle must pass medial to this vessel; laceration of the artery is the main complication of this route.

Complications

- Vasovagal reaction (bradycardia, hypotension)
- Arrhythmias
- Laceration of heart
- Laceration of coronary arteries
- Pneumothorax and laceration of the lung
- Laceration of the internal mammary artery
- Spread of infection from a purulent effusion

Aftercare

The patient should remain on the ECG monitor for two hours after the procedure with observation of clinical condition, pulse, and blood pressure every 15 minutes. Any complication of the procedure is likely to manifest within this period. A repeat echocardiogram and chest radiograph are strongly recommended. Both should be carried out at the bedside.

Interpretation of the results

- If tamponade is the cause of haemodynamic embarrassment, clinical improvement may rapidly be observed after drawing off only 200–300 ml fluid.
- An increasingly blood stained effusion is a sign of needle trauma, so preserve the earliest specimens for cell count and biochemistry. Later samples can be used for culture.
- A haemorrhagic aspiration is often present in malignant effusion and is to be expected in trauma.

Guard against troubleshooting

To minimise the risk of complications, bear the following points in mind:

- The smaller the effusion, the more difficult and hazardous the procedure. For elective aspiration, there should be at least 1 cm of free pericardial space
- Stopcock reduces the risk of pneumothorax should the needle enter the pleural space
- Lateral "lacerating" movement of the needle should be avoided. If change of direction is required, withdraw the needle and insert again in the new direction
- Appearance of ectopic beats is an indication for partial withdrawal of the needle, but the direction is usually correct
- Two dimensional echocardiographic guidance is not essential in most cases, but can be valuable in aspiration of loculated effusions
- In a severely distressed patient with documented tamponade, but in whom immediate aspiration cannot be performed, administration of intravenous fluids may delay haemodynamic deterioration. This is no replacement for urgent aspiration which should be performed as soon as possible
- Raised jugular venous pressure in a breathless patient may increase the temptation to administer diuretics, especially because oliguria is a common feature of tamponade. Diuretics and vasodilators may precipitate circulatory collapse and should be avoided

Part II
Medical diagnosis and therapy

10 Lumbar puncture

JMS PEARCE

Indications

Lumbar puncture should not be indulged in idly as a result of diagnostic bankruptcy or in place of a neurological opinion. Though it may be informative in certain patients with coma or stroke it should not be done blindly as an immediate procedure until other diagnostic tests have been performed.

There are three main indications:

1. For diagnostic purposes (Box A).
2. For introducing contrast media.
3. For introducing chemotherapeutic agents – for example, in meningitis or leukaemia.

Contraindications

Contraindications are the following:

- *Raised intracranial pressure*, indicated by morning or postural headache, vomiting, and papilloedema: even in the absence of signs, a history suspicious of increased pressure contraindicates lumbar puncture and should lead to a neurological consultation and computed tomography. The danger exists of fatal transtentorial or cerebellar "coning".
- *Suspected cord compression*: in many isolated cord lesions it is not possible to distinguish an intrinsic lesion (for example, multiple sclerosis) from extrinsic compression by disc or tumour.

111

Box A   Indications for lumbar puncture

Indications	Tests
Diagnostic	
Suspected subarachnoid haemorrhage if CT or MRI are negative or equivocal	Uniform blood staining, xanthochromia
Selected strokes, but not routinely	Red cells, protein
Myelopathies and suspected multiple sclerosis, but not for suspected cord compression	Cells, protein, immunoglobulins, oligoclonal bands
Peripheral neuropathies – for example, Guillain–Barré syndrome	Cells, protein, immunology, and microbiology
Infections of central nervous system(bacterial meningitis; tuberculosis; acute and subacute encephalitides; neurosyphilis; viral, fungal, and protozoal meningitis: especially in immunocompromised or HIV positive patients	Cells, protein, glucose, culture, virology. Tuberculosis and haemophilus antigens, treponemal haemagglutinins (or other specific treponemal tests). Other special stains and antibodies, for example, Indian ink stain or antigen for torulosis; anti-HIV-I IgG in HIV encephalopathy
Radiology	
Introduction of contrast media	
Therapeutic	
Introduction of antibiotics or opioids in selected cases	
Removal of CSF in benign intracranial hypertension	

Diagnostic lumbar puncture does not resolve this problem. Myelography with simultaneous cerebrospinal fluid examination and computed tomography or magnetic resonance imaging are the investigations of choice.

● *Local sepsis*: puncture through infected skin carries the risk of meningitis; lumbar puncture must be avoided.

Procedure

The most important factor in achieving an easy lumbar puncture is the correct positioning of the patient. The procedure should be explained to the patient and he or she should be comfortable and relaxed.

Place the patient on the left side with his or her back right up against the edge of the bed or firm trolley. Both legs are flexed towards the chest: place a pillow between the legs to ensure that the back is vertical. The neck should be slightly flexed (Fig 1).

Mask and gloves should be worn. Clean the skin with iodine and spirit (or other antiseptic) and then position the sterile drapes. Use a 22–25 small gauge needle if possible to avoid a large hole in the dura; in a rigid "arthritic spine" a larger, 18–20 gauge needle will sometimes prove necessary. When using the needle try to keep the bevel in the vertical, axial plane of the dural fibres, thus minimising the size of the hole.

Palpate the anterosuperior iliac spine. The interspace perpendicularly beneath it is that at L3–L4. As the spinal cord ends at L1–L2 the spaces above and below L3–L4 are equally acceptable sites. Palpate the spinous processes superior to the chosen interspace: the needle will be inserted about 1 cm inferior to the tip of the process.

Draw up 5 ml 2% plain lignocaine and, stretching the skin evenly over the interspace, infiltrate the skin and deeper tissues.

Allow at least one minute for the lignocaine to work, then introduce the needle. Make sure that the needle is 90° to the back,

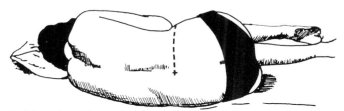

FIG 1   Left lateral position for lumbar puncture, usually between L3 and L4; the back should be perpendicular to the horizontal axis of the bed or couch, the needle in the midline, pointed slightly towards the head

with its bevel in the sagittal plane and pointing slightly to the head. Push the needle through the resistance of the superficial supraspinous ligament. The interspinous ligament is then easily negotiated. At about 4–7 cm the firmer resistance of the ligamentum flavum is felt, when an extra push will result in a popping sensation as the dura is breached.

The needle should now lie in the subarachnoid space and, when the stylet is withdrawn, clear colourless fluid should drip out (Fig 2).

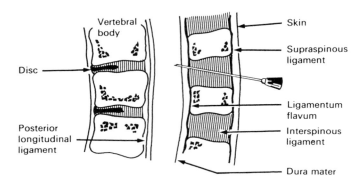

FIG 2 Needle insertion through L3–L4 interspinous ligament penetrates the ligamentum flavum. The resistance to insertion lessens as the dura is penetrated and CSF flows

Dry tap

If no fluid emerges or it does not flow easily rotate the needle, because a flap of dura may be lying against the bevel. If there is still no fluid reinsert the stylet and cautiously advance, withdrawing the stylet after each movement. Pain radiating down either leg indicates that the needle is too lateral and has hit nerve roots. Withdraw the needle almost completely, check the patient's position, and reinsert in the midline (Fig 3).

If the needle meets total obstruction do not force it as the needle may be lying against an intervertebral disc and could damage it. Again, withdraw the needle, check its position, and reinsert. If there is complete failure move one space up or down depending on the original position. The procedure may be easier if the patient is sitting up.

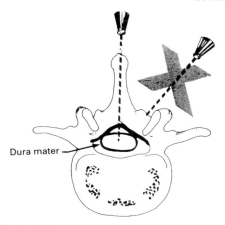

Dura mater

FIG 3 The needle should be inserted in the midline. If inserted laterally, the posterior facet joints and pedicle will impede puncture of the dura

A dry tap is usually the result of a failure of technique. After two or three attempts a colleague should be invited to show his or her superior skill. Rare causes of a genuine dry tap are arachnoiditis and infiltrations of the meninges.

Manometry

When the cerebrospinal fluid (CSF) flows freely the pressure should be measured. A manometer is connected to the hub of the needle directly or through a two way tap. An assistant holds the top end and pressure is recorded (normal 80–180 mm CSF (0·78–1·76 kPa)) (Fig 4). The height of the meniscus should be seen to change with respiration. Pressure on the jugular veins should cause a rise of >40 mm CSF (0·392 kPa) pressure (a negative Queckenstedt's test), but this has been replaced by magnetic resonance imaging or computed tomographic myelography if obstruction of the spinal canal is suspected.

Spinal block causes a failure of free rise and fall (positive Queckenstedt) and is usually accompanied by yellowish CSF with a high protein content (Froin's syndrome).

The most common cause of low CSF pressure is bad needle placement, but if the low pressure is genuine no attempt should be made to aspirate as the cause may be obstruction of CSF flow

115

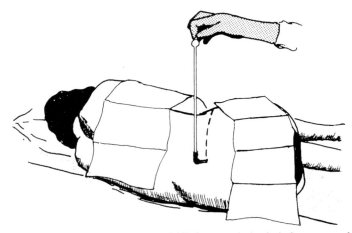

FIG 4 Needle in correct position: CSF flows and the hub is connected to a manometer held in the vertical plane to read the CSF pressure, and change with respiration, abdominal compression, and jugular venous compression

caused by cerebellar tonsil herniation or spinal block. In either case a neurological opinion is needed urgently.

A slightly raised CSF pressure in a very anxious or fat patient may be ignored. Pressures > 250 mm CSF (2·45 kPa) are abnormal and should be investigated. If a greatly raised pressure is discovered in a clear fluid the CSF should be collected from the manometer and the needle withdrawn. The patient should be nursed flat and a neurologist or neurosurgeon consulted.

Specimens for diagnosis

Samples (8–10 ml) of CSF are collected (Fig 5). The minimal requirements are a record of opening pressure, total and differential cell count, and total protein. There are no other routine tests and additional studies are dictated by the clinical queries and by close liaison with the local laboratories. Glucose is unnecessary unless an infective or neoplastic meningitis is considered; Lange curves, Pandy tests, and chlorides are obsolete.

A ward specimen of 1 ml is useful in suspected subarachnoid bleeding, in which xanthochromia (a yellow discoloured supernatant) may be observed before the laboratory report. It may also be a useful spare for "mislaid specimens".

Box B   Some CSF profiles

Purulent: high WBC, mainly polymorphs, low glucose ±

Infections
    Bacterial meningitis, viral meningitis (early)
    TB meningitis (early)
    Cerebral abscess, subdural empyema, intracranial thrombo-
      phlebitis

Non-infectious
Chemical meningitis (for example, after contrast media)
    Mollaret's recurrent meningitis

Lymphocytic: high WBC, mainly lymphocytes, low glucose

Infections
    TB, fungal, treponemal, leptospiral, listeria, and half treated
      bacterial meningitis
    Viral meningitis

Non-infectious
    Carcinomatous, lymphomatous, leukaemic "meningitis"
    Sarcoidosis

Lymphocytic: high WBC, mainly lymphocytes, normal glucose

Infections
    Viral meningitis, encephalitis (for example, herpes simplex)
    Half treated bacterial meningitis
    Parameningeal infections (abscess, intracranial
      thrombophlebitis)
    Fungal and TB meningitis (early)
    Parasitic infestation (for example, trichinosis, toxoplasmosis,
      amoebiasis)
    HIV-1 nervous system infections*

Non-infectious
    Post-infectious encephalitis, myelitis
    Acute demyelination (MS)

*Glucose normal or slightly decreased.

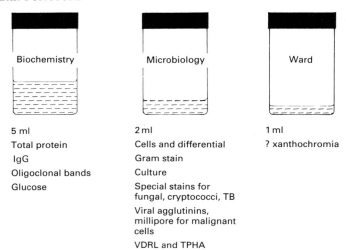

Biochemistry	Microbiology	Ward
5 ml	2 ml	1 ml
Total protein	Cells and differential	? xanthochromia
IgG	Gram stain	
Oligoclonal bands	Culture	
Glucose	Special stains for fungal, cryptococci, TB	
	Viral agglutinins, millipore for malignant cells	
	VDRL and TPHA	

FIG 5 CSF is collected in three bottles as shown, and sent to laboratories for analysis. VDRL, Venereal Disease Reference Laboratory test; TPHA, *Treponema pallidum* haemagglutination test

Even the most careful lumbar puncture can be bedevilled by blood staining. Bloody fluid should be collected in three tubes. A traumatic tap can be distinguished from subarachnoid haemorrhage in three ways:

1. Blood resulting from trauma forms streams in an otherwise clear CSF, whereas the CSF of subarachnoid bleeding is diffusely blood stained.

2. On centrifugation or standing the supernatant is colourless in a traumatic tap but xanthochromic in subarachnoid haemorrhage. The only exception is that a clear supernatant may rarely occur if the lumbar puncture is done within six hours of a subarachnoid haemorrhage occurring.

3. The first three consecutive specimens of CSF in a traumatic tap show clearing of the blood and usually become colourless, with a corresponding fall of the red cell count in the third bottle.

Aftercare and complications

Once the specimens have been collected, the needle is removed. The patient may be nursed flat, prone, or tilted head down for 24 hours, but it is debatable whether this hallowed routine lessens the incidence of headache. Headache after lumbar puncture is a low intracranial pressure state resulting from persistent leakage of CSF through the hole(s) in the dura. Prevention demands a careful technique and the use of a small gauge needle. Headache occurs in about 10–20% of patients and may be accompanied by vomiting. It is treated by laying the patient flat, bed tilted head down, and by the liberal use of analgesics (aspirin, paracetamol, or codeine phosphate) with antiemetics (metoclopramide or domperidone) (Fig 6). It usually lasts 36–72 hours, but may occasionally persist for a week. The onset may be delayed for three or four days. A similar picture occurs after spinal anaesthetic; many anaesthetists use an "epidural blood patch" to prevent or treat this condition.

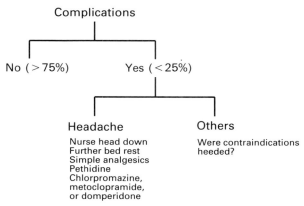

FIG 6   Complications of lumbar puncture

Interpretation of results

Cerebrospinal fluid

Findings in neurological disease are given in Table I. Normal values are given in Table II.

CSF findings should always be interpreted in the light of clinical features and other laboratory results. A raised CSF protein always implies a lesion of the CNS but is itself seldom diagnostic.

119

TABLE I Typical CSF findings in neurological diseases

Pathology	CSF	WBC (/mm³)	Protein (g/l)	Glucose (mmol/l)
Normal	Clear and colourless	0–5	0·15–0·45	2·7–4·5 (60% blood glucose)
Subarachnoid haemorrhage	Bloody with xantho-chromia	5000 RBCs + WBCs 0–100	0·4–1·0	2·7–4·5
Multiple sclerosis	Clear and colourless	Lymphocytes 0–100	0·15–1·0 IgG + oligo-clonal bands	2·7–4·5
Spinal block (Froin's syndrome)	Yellow	0–5	2–10	2·7–4·5
Bacterial meningitis	Turbid or purulent	1000–10 000	0·5–1·5	0–3·0
		85% + polymorphonuclears		
Viral meningitis	Clear	50–1000 mixed* early → mainly lymphocytes	0·15–1·2	2·7–4·5
Fungal meningitis	Purulent or cloudy	100–1000 mixed*, mainly lymphocytes ± fungal bodies	0·5–1·5	0·1–4·5
Tuberculous meningitis	Clear or opalescent with web	5–500 mixed* early → lymphocytes	0·4–1·5	0–4·0
General paralysis of the insane, neurosyphilis	Clear	5–500 lymphocytes	0·5–1·2 IgG + oligoclonal bands and TPHA	2·7–4·5

* Mixed pleocytosis, 30–70% polymorphonuclears, remainder monocytes.

TABLE II Some normal values for CSF

		Diagnostic value
Opening pressure	50–180 mm CSF (0·49–1·76 kPa)	Raised intracranial pressure
Osmolarity	29·5 mosmol/l*	Rarely
pH	7·31*	Rarely
Total WBCs	0–5/mm^3	Inflammatory states
Total protein	0·15–0·45 g/l	Non-specific (immune or demyelinating diseases)
γ Globulin	3–12% of total	
IgG	<0·06 g/l	
Glucose	2–4·5 mmol/l	Pyogenic, fungal, TB, malignant infiltrations
VDRL, TPHA, TPI	Negative	Syphilis
Lactate	1·6 mmol/l*	Pyogenic meningitis
Ammonia	300 µg/l*	Hepatic encephalopathy
		Reye's syndrome

* Average values.
VDRL, Venereal Disease Research Laboratory test; TPHA, *Treponema pallidum* haemagglutination test; TPI, *Treponema pallidum* immobilisation test. WBC, white blood cell count; TB, tuberculosis.

11 Pleural aspiration and biopsy

PB ILES
S KUMAR

Indications

Pleural aspiration is an important diagnostic procedure and is often used therapeutically to relieve dyspnoea caused by large effusions or to instil agents such as cytotoxics or sclerosants into the pleural space. It can prevent effusions – especially those that are purulent or haemorrhagic – from becoming chronic and thus avoid the development of pleural thickening and a "frozen" chest. Pleural biopsy should normally be combined with the first aspiration because this increases the diagnostic yield and there may be insufficient pleural fluid remaining on later occasions to permit a safe biopsy.

In instances where the aetiology of an effusion can be reasonably deduced from clinical grounds (for example, heart failure) the procedure can be deferred and the response to therapy observed.

Special precautions

It may be hazardous to perform a pleural biopsy when clotting is impaired and, if possible, this should be corrected before the procedure. There are increased risks with small effusions especially if patients have underlying chronic lung disease (such as severe chronic obstructive airway disease). There is a recognised risk of seeding mesothelioma cells in the biopsy track and, therefore, if this disease is suspected from the clinical features, it is wise to reserve biopsy for those patients in whom pleural fluid cytology has not been diagnostic. Chest wall infection and inability of the patient to cooperate are also relative contraindications.

Equipment

Diagnostic pleural aspiration
    Sterile gloves, gown, and towels
    Dressing pack
    Skin antiseptic
    Syringes: 10 ml and 50 ml
    Hypodermic needles
    Specimen bottles

For therapeutic aspiration
    As above
    Lignocaine 1% or 2%
    Intravenous cannulas: 14 gauge or 17 gauge (length 45 mm)
    Three way tap with rubber or plastic tubing
    Receiver for fluid
    Adhesive dressing

Pleural biopsy
    As above
    Scalpel blade (fine pointed)
    Abram's needle
    Suture pack

Aspiration procedure

Before you start, review the most recent posteroanterior and lateral chest radiographs and re-examine the patient to decide the most appropriate site for the procedure. If in doubt about whether there is an effusion or consolidation, ultrasonography should resolve the uncertainty and also determine the best site for aspiration.

It is important that the patient is as comfortable and relaxed as possible. Full explanation of the procedure should be given. The patient should be positioned leaning slightly forward with the arms folded comfortably and resting on a pillow, placed on a support such as a bed table. When the fluid is not loculated, the easiest site for puncture is the posterior chest wall medial to the angle of the scapula, one interspace below the upper limit of dullness to percussion. The operator should scrub up and be gloved and gowned as for any other invasive procedure. The patient's skin is prepared with a suitable antiseptic and sterile towels. For a diagnostic aspiration, local anaesthesia is usually unnecessary because sufficient fluid can be obtained at a single pass. If large volumes are to be aspirated, local anaesthesia is used. The skin overlying an intercostal space at the chosen level is infiltrated with 1% or 2% lignocaine using a 25 gauge (orange hub) needle. This is then changed for a 21 gauge (green hub) needle to infiltrate the chest wall down to the pleura. When the needle penetrates the pleura, fluid should appear in the syringe as the plunger is withdrawn. To avoid damaging the intercostal neurovascular bundle, the inferior border of the upper rib should be avoided.

For a diagnostic tap, 50 ml of fluid is usually aspirated. In a non-obese subject, a 21 gauge venepuncture needle with 50 ml syringe is inserted perpendicularly to the chest wall (Figs 1 and 2). In obese patients or if the pleura is felt to be greatly thickened, a long lumbar puncture needle may be used.

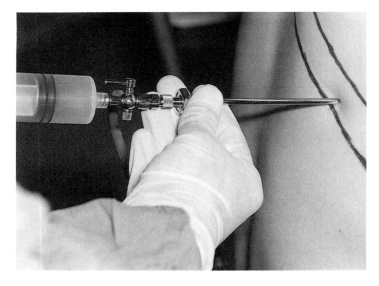

FIG 1   Aspiration using Abram's needle. The rib interspace has been outlined

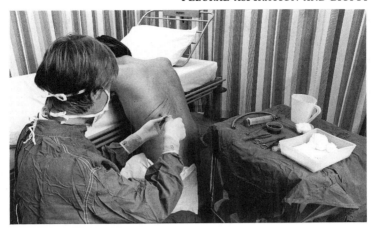

FIG 2   Pleural aspirator

Samples are routinely sent for estimation of protein concentration, differential cell count, cytology, and microbiology. Occasionally fluid is sent for amylase, serology, pH, and lactate dehydrogenase measurements.

When aspirating large volumes of fluid, it is easier and safer to insert an intravenous cannula. After infiltrating local anaesthetic, the cannula with a 10 ml syringe attached is gently inserted until fluid is aspirated. The needle is pulled out approximately 1 cm and the cannula is pushed in further until it is in apposition to the chest wall (this avoids buckling of the plastic cannula when aspirating). The needle is then completely removed and a closed three way tap attached. Fluid is aspirated using a 50 ml syringe. Care must be taken to ensure that air does not enter the pleural space at any stage of the procedure. When the cannula is removed, a small adhesive dressing is applied at the puncture site.

Failure to obtain any fluid may result from insertion of the needle too low down or too far forward. If uncertain try higher. If the pleura feels unusually thick and the needle moves through a wide arc on respiration, it is probably in the diaphragm. If only a small quantity of fluid is obtained, the collection may be loculated. No fluid may be present, for example, if there is consolidation or marked pleural thickening. The value of ultrasonography in identifying fluid in these instances has been discussed.

125

Patients with empyema and haemothorax

Difficulties may arise in patients with empyema and haemothorax when the fluid is thick and loculated. Aspiration may be possible only with a large bore needle and exploratory aspiration at several sites may be necessary (ultrasonography may help). Repeated aspiration should be continued until pus is no longer obtained. If there is still evidence of continuing infection, insertion of an intercostal drainage tube is advisable. The decision regarding tube drainage is an important one, because delay may permit further organisation of the fibropurulent exudate, necessitating later open surgical drainage or decortication. In parapneumonic effusions, pleural fluid pH measurements are helpful in the decision to place a chest drain – a fall in pH precedes the appearance of organisms in the fluid and suggests the need for tube drainage.

Intrapleural instillation of antibiotics is seldom required these days because of increased tissue penetration of newer antibiotics. Uniformly blood stained fluid which does not clot suggests a haemothorax. If uncertain it is valuable to measure the haematocrit. Tube drainage is usually indicated in haemothorax.

Biopsy equipment

The Abram's needle is the most widely used in Britain for pleural biopsy (Fig 3). A Tru-Cut needle (which produces similar results to Abram's needle) can also be used, but is usually reserved for pleural masses or lung biopsy. The Abram's needle consists of outer and inner tubes, the outer acting as a trocar. Behind the lip of

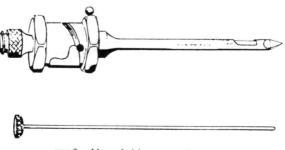

FIG 3 Abram's biopsy needle

the outer tube there is an opening into which a fold of pleura is impacted. This opening is closed completely when the cutting edge of the inner tube is advanced by twisting its hexagonal grip clockwise. This rotation moves a pin in the hilt of the inner tube forwards along a spiral slot in the hilt of the outer tube. The biopsy specimen is cut by a sharp advancing edge of the inner tube and is retained within the instrument. It can then be retrieved by using the accompanying blunt obturator.

Biopsy technique

Position and prepare the patient as for a pleural aspiration and infiltrate the intercostal tissues at the chosen site generously with lignocaine. It is important to check that fluid can be aspirated into the syringe. Note also the approximate thickness of the chest wall down to the pleura. Make a stab incision through the skin and subcutaneous tissue. The closed Abram's needle is then introduced through the tissues. The temptation to push in an uncontrolled manner must be resisted. Firm pressure is exerted with the dominant hand, while gripping the needle barrel approximately 2 cm from the tip with the other hand. The parietal pleura is penetrated with a slight rotatory movement of the needle. The hand on the barrel acts to prevent the needle suddenly penetrating too deeply. The needle is normally air tight when the notch is closed but a syringe or closed three way tap must be attached when the notch is open to prevent air entering the pleural cavity. Rotate the hexagonal hub on the inner tube anti-clockwise to open the notch and aspirate pleural fluid in the usual manner (Fig 4).

When taking a biopsy specimen, rotate the grip to open the notch, which faces the same direction as the spherical marker on one facet of the hexagonal hub of the outer tube. With this marker (and therefore the notch) facing along the line of the intercostal space, apply lateral pressure towards the notch with the forefinger and slowly withdraw the needle until resistance is felt owing to the pleura catching in the notch. If the needle is withdrawn too far only intercostal muscle will be biopsied. Hold the needle firmly and sharply twist the grip of the inner tube clockwise to take the specimen. Withdraw the needle with a slight rotatory action when the patient exhales, covering the entry site with a gauze swab as the needle emerges. To avoid damage to the intercostal neurovascular

127

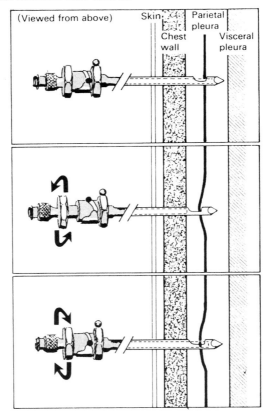

FIG 4   Pleural biopsy with Abram's needle

bundle, the notch should *never* be directed upwards. The specimen will be found either within the inner tube or in the tip of the needle and should be put in formalin. It is advisable to take three or four specimens if possible. If tuberculous pleurisy is suspected, some of the pleural biopsy specimens should be placed in saline for bacteriological culture.

Complications

It is wise to obtain a chest radiograph after pleural aspiration, particularly if any difficulty was experienced (for example, air

128

drawn back into the syringe) or a large volume of fluid aspirated. It is essential after pleural biopsy or if the patient experiences chest tightness or bouts of coughing. Pneumothorax can result if the needle tip penetrates the visceral pleura or if air is inadvertently allowed to enter via the needle. Pneumothorax is estimated to occur in 3–20% of patients, of whom 20% may require chest tube insertion.

If fluid is removed too quickly or in too large a quantity, oedema may develop in the re-expanded lung tissue. It is usually recommended that not more than 1·0–1·5 litres is aspirated at one time, although in small patients even 700 ml may be the limit. If the lung is unable to re-expand freely, a high negative intrapleural pressure may develop as fluid is aspirated. This will be felt by the operator as an increased pull on the syringe plunger and by the patient as chest tightness accompanied by coughing. This complication can be relieved by letting air into the pleural space to lower the negative pressure, but this delays re-expansion of the lung and may permit loculation of the fluid. In the absence of a clotting defect pleural aspiration rarely leads to serious haemoptysis or haemothorax. The former may occur if pleural biopsy is attempted without first obtaining fluid and the latter if the vessels at the lower border of the rib are damaged.

If the aspiration needle tears the visceral pleura and a superficial vein, air may be sucked into the pulmonary veins from the needle itself or from adjacent lung. The air may enter any systemic artery, most often the cerebral vessels, and produce transient neurological symptoms and signs. The customary emergency treatment is to tilt the patient's head down and with the right side uppermost to reduce the chance of air entering these arteries. Many deaths previously certified as "pleural shock" were probably the result of air embolus, but vagal inhibition can also occur. Empyema is rare, but nevertheless infection may be introduced especially if strict aseptic technique is not properly adhered to. Other possible complications are tumour seeding in cases of mesothelioma and biopsy of other viscera.

Thoracoscopy

This technique has usually been performed under general anaesthesia by thoracic surgeons but has now also been practised by

TABLE I Interpretation of results

Condition	Appearance	Pleural : serum protein ratio	Cells	Cytology	Biopsy	Other features
Secondary to infection	Clear or cloudy	>0·5	Polymorphs +	Negative	Inflammatory reaction, fibrinous exudate, or fibrosis	
Empyema	Cloudy or purulent	>0·5	Polymorphs + + +	Negative	Inflammatory reaction, fibrinous exudate, or fibrosis	*Staphylococcus aureus* *Streptococcus pneumoniae* Anaerobes pH <7·2
Tuberculosis	Clear or cloudy	>0·5	Lymphocytes + or + +	Negative	Granuloma in 60%	Biopsy culture positive in 90%
Secondary to malignancy	Bloody or clear	>0·5	Lymphocytes +	Positive in 50%	Positive in 45%	70% positive when cytology and histology combined

Mesothelioma	Bloody	>0·5	Mesothelial cells	Positive in 25–50%	Positive in 40–60%	Special stains required
Pulmonary infarction	Bloody or clear	Variable	Red blood cells Polymorphs Eosinophils	Negative	Non-specific	
Hypoproteinaemia/ cardiac failure	Clear	<0·5	Usually none	Negative	Negative	
Connective tissue disease	Clear or cloudy	>0·5	Lymphocytes	Negative	Non-specific	SLE ANF +ve LE cells present Rheumatoid arthritis RF +ve LDH high Glucose low

SLE, systemic lupus erythematosus; ANF, anti-nuclear factor; LE, lupus erythematosus; RF, rheumatoid factor; LDH, lactate dehydrogenase.

physicians under local anaesthesia using a fibreoptic bronchoscope instead of a rigid thoracoscope. Details of the method are beyond the scope of this chapter, but it is the most reliable method of obtaining a positive pleural biopsy specimen.

Interpretation of results

The pattern of results seen most frequently is given in the table; inevitably it is incomplete. The following points are worth remembering. Pleural effusions are generally divided into transudates and exudates. Transudates are the result of alterations in hydrostatic pressure or decreased oncotic pressure. Traditionally effusions with pleural protein > 30 g/l were classified as exudates, but if this criterion is used solely, some exudates will be classified erroneously as transduates. Of exudates 99% (and transudates none) have at least one of the characteristics shown in the box.

- Pleural fluid protein:serum protein ratio > 0.5
- Pleural fluid lactate dehydrogenase (LDH):serum ratio > 0.6
- Pleural fluid LDH more than two thirds of the upper limit of normal for serum LDH (200 international units/litre or IU/l)

Pleural exudates are most commonly malignant, followed in frequency by those resulting from infections. Pulmonary infarction is an important consideration in any undiagnosed pleural effusion. Immunological diseases (systemic lupus erythematosus, rheumatoid arthritis) are associated with pleural effusions, rarely as the only initial manifestation of the disease. Tuberculous pleurisy should always be considered as a differential diagnosis, in which case pleural biopsy should be sent for culture as well as histological investigation.

12 Abdominal paracentesis

A HIGHAM
A WATSON

In the first half of this century, abdominal paracentesis was a common therapeutic procedure in patients with ascites. Following the introduction of effective diuretic therapy and publications in the 1950s describing the potential hazards of such intervention, abdominal paracentesis fell from favour. More recent research has demonstrated therapeutic abdominal paracentesis to be effective and safe for the rapid relief and control of large volume ascites. This article discusses the indications and practicalities of performing abdominal paracentesis, and in particular therapeutic paracentesis for large volume ascites caused by chronic liver disease.

Detection of ascites

At least 500 ml free intraperitoneal fluid must be present before the clinical sign of shifting dullness becomes apparent, and considerably more before a fluid thrill is detectable. Large volume ascites will produce distension of the flanks and abdominal wall, and, if longstanding, umbilical and other abdominal hernias. The clinical signs of ascites may be misinterpreted (for example, in the presence of distended and fluid filled loops of intestine) and, if in doubt, ultrasonography is the investigation of choice for confirming the presence of ascites. As little as 100 ml free fluid within the peritoneum may be detected by ultrasonography and therefore may be found incidentally. Nevertheless, once detected further investigation is warranted as ascites always indicates serious underlying disease.

Diagnostic paracentesis

Abdominal paracentesis as a diagnostic investigation is a simple and a safe procedure. It is mandatory in patients with ascites either presenting for the first time, where the cause is unknown or in any patient in whom infected ascites is a possibility. Contraindications to performing diagnostic paracentesis blind are few and relative. They include multiple previous operations, clinically obvious intestinal distension, and pregnancy. In these circumstances ultrasonic guidance is prudent.

Procedure

The patient's informed consent should be obtained and his or her bladder should be empty. For diagnostic purposes 60 ml fluid usually suffices and less if exclusion of infection is the only objective. The necessary equipment is shown in Box A.

Box A   Equipment necessary for diagnostic and therapeutic paracentesis

Diagnostic paracentesis
- Dressing pack
- Skin disinfection
- 10 ml syringe with 23 + 19 gauge needles
- 1% lignocaine
- 60 ml syringe with 16 gauge needle
- Specimen containers
- Sterile gloves

Therapeutic paracentesis (in addition to the above)
- Face mask and gown
- Sterile towels
- Trocar and cannula
- Collection system
- Scalpel and blade
- Suture pack and sutures
- Intravenous giving set and plasma expander

The patient lies semi-recumbent and is examined to determine the puncture site. This should demonstrate dullness to percussion and avoid solid organs and underlying large vessels (Fig 1). The iliac fossae are most often used. The patient may need to roll slightly to the chosen side to maximise the area of dullness, and then the chosen site is marked. The operator should wash, put on sterile gloves, and disinfect the puncture site. After this, the skin, subcutaneous tissue, muscle layers, and peritoneum are infiltrated

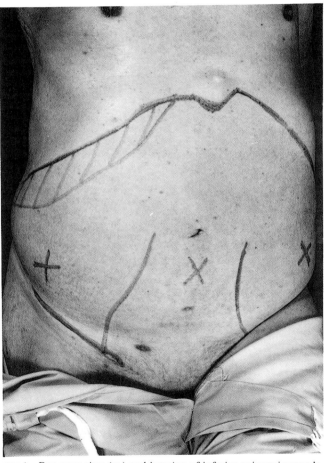

FIG 1   Puncture sites (×) and location of inferior epigastric vessels

with local anaesthetic. The needle tract should be oblique to minimise post-puncture leaking. With the 60 ml syringe attached, the 16 gauge needle is introduced along the anaesthetised tract into the peritoneal cavity and 50–60 ml fluid withdrawn. Following the procedure a simple dry dressing is applied.

Potential problems

The only common problem is a "dry" tap. This may indicate failure to enter the peritoneum, perforation of a viscus, occlusion of the needle by omentum, or absence of ascites. A further attempt following repositioning of the needle and/or the patient is reasonable. If this fails an inexperienced operator should consider seeking help from a more experienced colleague. If no fluid can be obtained then ultrasonography should be requested to confirm ascites and guide future attempts at paracentesis.

Investigations

The ascites should be inspected because its appearance may suggest the underlying pathology. Fluid (10 ml) should be sent for measurement of protein concentration and amylase concentration if necessary. The remainder should be sent for cytology, white cell count, microscopy, and culture. The results of the investigations are most helpful when interpreted in the context of the full clinical presentation. A summary and interpretation of laboratory results for the more common causes of ascites are shown in the table.

Therapeutic paracentesis

Therapeutic paracentesis is once again gaining acceptance as a simple procedure for the rapid relief and control of large volume ascites. In selected patients the procedure is as safe as diuretic therapy, provided appropriate precautions are taken, including the administration of a suitable plasma volume expander to compensate for the hypovolaemic effect of the drainage. Therapeutic paracentesis reduces inpatient hospital stay; one recent study demonstrated that therapeutic paracentesis required a hospital stay of 11 days compared to 31 days for diuretic therapy. Nevertheless, it should be stressed that most patients with ascites can and should be managed initially with dietary salt restriction and diuretic therapy.

Summary of laboratory investigations for the more common causes of ascites

Source of ascites	Appearance	Protein concn (g/l)	White cell count (× 10⁹/l)	Microscopy	Culture
Uncomplicated cirrhosis	Clear	<30	<0·3 (>75% lymphocytes)	Negative	Negative
Neoplasia	Blood stained or clear	>30*	0·1–1·0	Positive cytology (usually)	Negative
Spontaneous bacterial peritonitis	Cloudy	>30*	>0·3 (>75% polymorphs)	Organisms often seen	Positive
Nephrotic syndrome	Clear	<20	<0·3 (>75% lymphocytes)	Negative	Negative
Tuberculosis	Clear/Cloudy	>30*	Variable (>50% lymphocytes)	Negative (usually)	Positive

* All are exudates and absolute protein concentration depends upon serum albumin.

137

Patient selection

The recent studies highlighting the benefits and safety of therapeutic paracentesis have been performed on selected patients. Until further evidence is presented to the contrary, large volume paracentesis should be restricted to similarly selected patients. Such intervention is therefore only indicated in the presence of massive or refractory ascites. Contraindications are shown in Box B.

Box B   Contraindications to therapeutic paracentesis

- Established hepatorenal failure
- Hepatic encephalopathy
- Sepsis
- Significant coagulopathy (international normalised ratio or INR $> 1 \cdot 4$, platelet count $< 40\,000/mm^3$)
- Gastrointestinal blood loss
- Serum $Na^+ < 125$ mmol/l
- Serum creatinine > 265 μmol/l
- Urinary sodium excretion > 10 mmol/day

Patient preparation

The patient should be admitted to hospital and his or her informed consent obtained. Diuretics should be stopped for 48 hours before the procedure and a careful fluid balance record kept. During this time all the remaining investigations should be completed to ensure that the necessary criteria for performing therapeutic paracentesis are fulfilled. Blood urea and electrolytes should be estimated on the day before the procedure.

Procedure

An intravenous cannula should be inserted so that administration of an appropriate plasma volume expander can be commenced once paracentesis begins. Puncture site selection and preparation of the patient should be as described above. Strict sterile precautions should be taken. Once the skin has been anaesthetised, a small stab incision should be made. Next a purse-string suture should be sited around the incision but not tied. The trocar and cannula (external diameter 2–3 mm) should then be advanced until they enter the peritoneal cavity. The patient should be asked to tense the abdominal muscles, which facilitates recognition of the sense of "give" as the peritoneal cavity is entered. The trocar is then removed, and the cannula advanced into the pelvis and attached to a drainage bag. The ascites should be allowed to flow freely until drainage ceases and the total volume of ascites measured. Intravenous administration of a plasma volume expander such as 20% salt poor albumin, Dextran 70, or gelatin should be commenced during drainage and be complete by 6 hours after the procedure. The authors' preference is to use gelatin (Haemaccel, Gelofusine) 150 ml for every litre of ascites, and to infuse half of the calculated volume as quickly as possible and complete the infusion over the remaining time. (For salt poor albumin 30 g/l ascites should be used and, for Dextran 70, 6 g/l ascites.) When the drainage of ascites is complete the intraperitoneal cannula should be removed, the purse-string suture tied and a dry dressing applied.

Post-procedure observations

Pulse rate and blood pressure should be recorded every half hour for the duration of the paracentesis and intravenous infusion, and hourly for the following 6 hours. A careful fluid balance record should be maintained. Patients should be assessed daily thereafter for probable complications of total paracentesis (Box C). Blood urea and electrolytes, together with full blood count, prothrombin time, and standard liver function tests, should be performed daily for the next two days, and for longer if any become deranged from those taken at baseline. Providing all the investigations remain unchanged diuretic therapy can be safely reinstituted 48 hours after the paracentesis. Any changes that do occur are usually apparent within 48 hours and generally return to baseline within seven days, although hyponatraemia may be more prolonged.

Complications

The reported complications are shown in Box C, the overall complication rates varying from approximately 13% to 33%. The most common complications are encephalopathy, renal impairment, and electrolyte disturbances. Encephalopathy and hyperkalaemia are usually readily reversible. In contrast, renal

---

Box C Estimated incidence of complications and adverse events from total therapeutic paracentesis

Complications	Incidence (%)
General	
Hyponatraemia	5–20
Encephalopathy	5–20
Renal impairment	0–5
Hyperkalaemia	0–5
Peritonitis	0–5
Local	
Wound infection	< 1
Abdominal wall oedema	< 1
Ascitic fluid leak	< 1
Other reported serious adverse events	
Gastrointestinal tract haemorrhage	5–15
Sepsis/bacteraemia	0–5

---

impairment tends to persist as does hyponatraemia in some patients. Peritonitis following the procedure is potentially life threatening but fortunately rare. Local complications such as an infected puncture site are also uncommon. Nevertheless, the complication rate of therapeutic paracentesis compares favourably with that of diuretic therapy. One recent study found the complication rates to be 17% *versus* 61% respectively, though no differences in survival were found.

Conclusion

Diagnostic paracentesis is a safe and simple procedure which is routinely performed and for which local expertise and guidance should be readily available. Therapeutic paracentesis is regaining acceptance as a useful adjunctive intervention for the control of large volume ascites. The procedure is as safe as diuretic therapy providing patients are carefully selected and appropriate precautions are taken.

Further reading

Gines P, Arroyo V, Quintero E, *et al*. Comparison of paracentesis and diuretics in the treatment of cirrhotics with tense ascites. *Gastroenterology* 1987; **93:** 234–41.

Gines P, Tito L, Arroyo V, *et al*. Randomised comparative study of therapeutic paracentesis with and without intravenous albumin in cirrhosis. *Gastroenterology* 1988; **94:** 1493–502.

Tito L, Gines P, Arroyo V, *et al*. Total paracentesis associated with intravenous albumin management of patients with cirrhosis and ascites. *Gastroenterology* 1990; **98:** 146–51.

Gines P, Arroyo V. Medical treatment of ascites. *Eur J Gastro Hepatol* 1991; **3:** 730–4.

13 Peritoneal dialysis

ER MAHER
JR CURTIS

Indications

Peritoneal dialysis is usually performed for acute or chronic renal failure, but may also be undertaken for pulmonary oedema, removal of toxins, hypothermia, and hypercalcaemia. When faced with a patient with renal failure you must first decide whether dialysis is necessary and then, if so, whether peritoneal dialysis or haemodialysis should be performed. General guidelines for dialysis in renal failure are hyperkalaemia (> 6.5 mmol/l), acidosis (pH < 7.1), urea > 40 mmol/l, or pulmonary oedema unresponsive to medical treatment. The advantages of peritoneal dialysis over haemodialysis are its relative simplicity and lack of life threatening complications. Peritoneal dialysis is preferred for patients with cardiovascular instability, for those in whom vascular access is difficult, and for those for whom anticoagulation would be hazardous.

Contraindications

Contraindications

- Recent abdominal surgery or trauma
- Extensive adhesions
- Ileostomy or colostomy
- Aortic vascular graft
- Inflammatory bowel disease
- Large intra-abdominal masses
- Indications for haemodialysis, such as hypoalbuminaemia or pulmonary insufficiency
- Large abdominal hernias

Most of these (see box) are relative contraindications, which increase the risk of catheter insertion or make peritoneal dialysis technically difficult.

Haemodialysis is more efficient than peritoneal dialysis and is preferred when rapid correction of electrolyte or fluid abnormalities is required. Other disadvantages of acute peritoneal dialysis are: immobility; loss of protein into the dialysate; metabolic disturbances (hyperglycaemia and hyperlipidaemia); and splinting of the diaphragm, reducing basal pulmonary ventilation. Haemodialysis is likely to be preferred for the treatment of hypercatabolic and malnourished patients or those with compromised pulmonary function, such as those requiring artificial ventilation. In acute renal failure, continuous arteriovenous (or venovenous) haemofiltration or continuous arteriovenous (or venovenous) haemodialysis is preferred for critically ill patients in intensive care units where patients are likely to be hypercatabolic and require artificial ventilation.

Chronic renal failure may be managed by intermittent haemodialysis, usually three times a week for 4–5 hours at a time, or by peritoneal dialysis which may be employed as continuous ambulatory peritoneal dialysis, usually with four exchanges daily, as intermittent peritoneal dialysis, or as continuous cycling peritoneal dialysis.

The ultimate choice of dialysis modality may be determined by local resources and availability.

Equipment

Many instruments are contained in an intravenous cut-down pack. We shall describe two methods of catheter insertion: one with a Trocath catheter and stylet unit and the second using a guide wire method. We favour the guide wire method as it is less traumatic and the catheter can be used for long term dialysis. The choice of method will depend on the physician's experience and the availability of catheters.

Before you start

- Obtain the consent of the patient.
- Ensure that the patient's bladder is empty (usually catheterisation is necessary).

Equipment

- Sterile gown, gloves, and mask
- Sterile surgical drapes
- Skin cleaning fluid
- Local anaesthetic
- 10 ml syringe, 21, 23, and 25 gauge needles
- 12 gauze swabs
- 16 gauge intravenous cannula
- Scalpel and no. 11 blade
- Scissors, skin stitch, and needle
- Catheter: Trocath stylet catheter unit or silicone peritoneal dialysis catheter (single or double cuff) with guide wire, introducer, and peelaway sheath (Fig 1)
- Peritoneal dialysis fluid (for example, 1·5% dextrose 1 litre bag and connecting set)
- 1 litre 0·9% NaCl and giving set

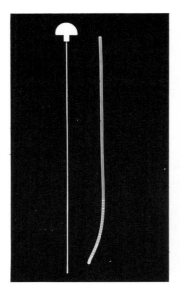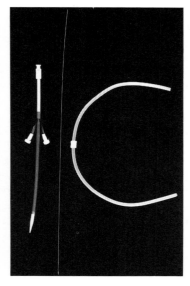

FIG 1   Two types of catheter: Trocath stylet–catheter unit (left) and single cuff silicone peritoneal dialysis catheter with guide wire, introducer, and peelaway sheath (right)

- Warm dialysis fluid and 1 litre 0·9% saline to body temperature.
- If necessary correct coagulation abnormalities before starting.

Procedure

General

1 Select a site for catheter insertion and clean skin with an iodine or chlorhexidine solution (Fig 2). The most common sites are in the midline, one third of the way from the umbilicus to the pubic symphysis (best site for the inexperienced), and in either iliac fossa level with the anterosuperior iliac spine about 2 cm lateral to the rectus sheath. Sites of surgical scars should be avoided.
2 Anaesthetise down to the peritoneum with 5 ml 2% lignocaine.
3 Make a small skin incision no wider than the diameter of the catheter.

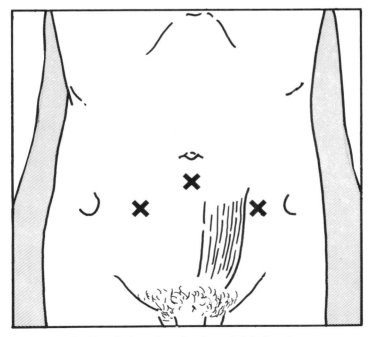

FIG 2   Sites for insertion of peritoneal dialysis catheters

145

4 Ask the patient (if conscious and cooperative) to tense his or her abdominal musculature (for example, by lifting the head against resistance). During this manoeuvre insert a 16 gauge intravenous cannula down to the peritoneum; there will be a slight give as you go through the peritoneum. Then advance the plastic sleeve and remove the needle. Infuse 1 litre of prewarmed 0·9% saline into the peritoneal cavity.

Trocath method

1 Remove the 16 gauge intravenous cannula. Then remove the plastic sleeve and insert the tip of the stylet–catheter unit through the skin incision.
2 Ask the patient to tense his or her abdomen again (see (4) above), and carefully push the stylet and catheter through the abdominal wall with a twisting action. As the peritoneum is punctured there is a sudden decrease in resistance. Excessive entry of the stylet may be prevented by holding the lower end of the stylet–catheter unit just above the skin.
3 On entering the peritoneal cavity, the stylet should be withdrawn 2–3 cm and the stylet and catheter advanced downwards into the pelvis at about 60° to the skin until about two thirds of the catheter have been inserted. The final part of the catheter is then advanced, as the stylet is withdrawn, until about 2 cm of catheter is left above the skin. The end of the catheter can then be attached to the connecting set to check that dialysis fluid will run in freely. If it does not, withdraw the catheter slightly and try again.
4 Put a purse-string suture around the catheter to prevent leakage, but do not overtighten.
5 Secure the catheter by pushing the metal disc over the catheter so that it lies against a gauze swab on the skin surface. Be careful not to bend the disc as then it will not retain the catheter. Trim the catheter so that 2 cm lie above the skin, and then reattach the connecting set. The L shaped connector should be supported in position by a wad of gauze to prevent kinking.

Guide wire method

1 Follow general steps (1)–(4) for the general method.
2 Insert a 0·038 inch (0·97 mm) guide wire through the intravenous cannula into the peritoneal cavity, then remove the

intravenous cannula. Use blunt dissection to make a small subcutaneous pocket for the Dacron cuff on the catheter.

3 Thread the introducer and peelaway sheath unit over the guide wire. Then ask the patient to tense his or her abdomen; push the introducer and sheath into the peritoneal cavity and direct it towards the pelvis. When the peelaway sheath is in position, withdraw the introducer and guide wire.

4 A single cuff soft silicone peritoneal dialysis catheter is then threaded through the sheath up to the level of the Dacron cuff. The outer sheath is then peeled away and the catheter advanced so that the cuff lies subcutaneously. A purse-string suture can be inserted as necessary.

5 In patients likely to need long term peritoneal dialysis, a double cuff Tenckhoff catheter can be inserted as above, except that a portion of the catheter is tunnelled so that the second cuff lies subcutaneously.

6 The catheter can then be attached to the peritoneal dialysis connecting line.

Problems

Problems
- Failure to drain
- Dialysate leakage
- Blood in dialysate

Failure to drain may be the result of a variety of causes. First, check the tubing is not kinked. If the catheter is blocked by fibrin flushing with heparin or urokinase may improve the flow. Treating constipation or changing the patient's position can also improve catheter function. If the catheter has been inserted into the preperitoneal space then failure to drain will be associated with swelling or oedema of the abdomen or scrotum. Radiographic examination of the abdomen will reveal whether the catheter is sited correctly in the pelvis. If the catheter is displaced from the pelvis or encased by omentum then the catheter must be re-positioned or replaced.

Dialysate leakage may be controlled by a purse string around the catheter or reducing the exchange volume.

Blood in dialysate usually clears after a few exchanges. Heparin (250 units/l) may be added to the dialysate to prevent clots blocking the catheter.

Complications

Bowel perforation is recognised by the presence of faecal material in the dialysate or the onset of Dextrostix positive watery diarrhoea. The catheter should be removed, antibiotics started – for example, metronidazole, cefuroxime, tobramycin – and a surgical opinion on laparotomy sought.

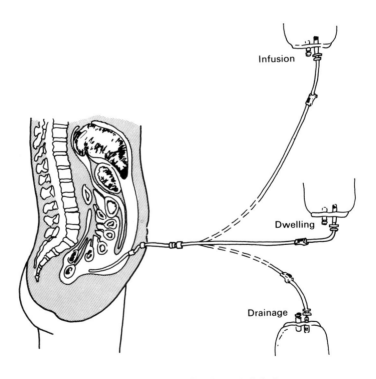

FIG 3   Technique of peritoneal dialysis

Peritonitis is usually caused by contamination during bag changes and so should be prevented by careful technique. It presents with cloudy bags and abdominal pain. Microscopy of the dialysate shows white cells and organisms. Intraperitoneal antibiotics (cefuroxime 200 mg/l and tobramycin 6 mg/l) are commenced until culture and sensitivities are available. Pain may be ameliorated by adding 10 ml 1% lignocaine to the dialysate.

Aftercare

Peritoneal dialysis (Fig 3) is commonly started with hourly 1 litre exchanges (10 min inflow, 30 min dwell, and 20 min outflow). If fluid removal is required every third or second exchange may be performed with a hypertonic bag (4·5% dextrose). Plasma potassium should be checked and potassium added to the dialysate bags as necessary. Hyperglycaemia may also occur, particularly if 4·5% dialysate is used. Trocath catheters should be replaced after 48 hours, but single or double cuff silicone catheters can be used for long term dialysis.

14 Bone marrow aspiration and trephine biopsy

AB MEHTA
AV HOFFBRAND

Bone marrow examination

Examination of the bone marrow is easily performed and carries a negligible risk of complications for the patient. It can provide essential diagnostic information about diseases arising primarily from within the bone marrow itself, and is also an accessible site for diagnosing diseases that have arisen elsewhere but have spread to involve the marrow. In addition to diagnosis, it also provides information on the extent of spread (stage) of malignant diseases. Examination of the bone marrow is essential for monitoring the effects of chemotherapy in patients with haematological malignancies and to assess grafting after bone marrow transplantation. The two methods of examination are bone marrow aspiration and trephine biopsy and indications for trephine biopsy are given in Table I. The needles for the two methods are shown in Figure 1.

Within the UK it is customary for clinical haematologists to perform the procedure themselves if they consider it appropriate after conducting a clinical assessment of the patient. The results of the peripheral blood count must be available, and the peripheral blood film should be examined as part of the clinical assessment.

Bone marrow aspiration

This is a less invasive procedure than trephine biopsy. Aspirated marrow is spread onto glass microscope slides (Fig 2) at the patient's bedside, and the slides are then stained and examined

150

TABLE 1 Indications for trephine biopsy

	Trephine biopsy		
	Optional	Recommended	Essential
Diagnosis			
Unexplained anaemia	+		
Thrombocytopenia	+		
Leucopenia	+		
Pancytopenia			+
Unexplained splenomegaly			+
Unexplained lymphadenopathy			+
Certain infections – for example, tuberculosis, leishmaniasis		+	
Suspected acute leukaemia		+	
Myelodysplasia		+	
Chronic leukaemia			+
Malignant lymphoma			+
Myeloproliferative disorders			+
Myeloma/macroglobinaemia		+	
Inherited disorders of intermediary metabolism – for example, lipid and glycogen storage disorders			+
Granulomatous diseases – for example, sarcoidosis			+
Staging			
Malignant lymphoma			+
Carcinoma			+
Monitoring therapy			
Acute leukaemia	+		
Myeloma	+		
Lymphoma			+
Bone marrow transplantation		+	

microscopically. The morphology of individual cells is well retained and the proportion of cells of different types is accurately assessed by counting at least 300 cells. Additional cytochemical stains may be used to characterise the cells further. Use of Perl's stain should be a routine procedure to assess iron stores and to detect abnormalities of iron use by developing erythroblasts – for example, lack of iron granules in iron deficiency or in the anaemia of chronic disorders, or rings of iron granules in sideroblastic anaemia. Cells may also be aspirated for other tests – for example,

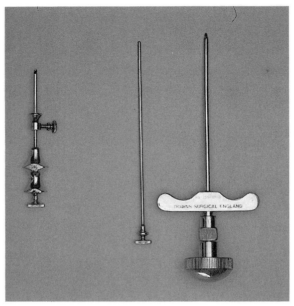

FIG 1 Islam bone marrow trephine needle (left) and Salah bone marrow aspirate needle (right)

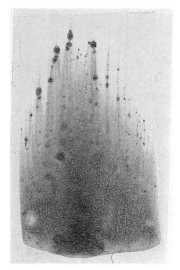

FIG 2 Bone marrow aspirate smeared on to a glass slide

microbiological culture, cytogenetic examination or specialised tests to characterise the disease process further (box).

Additional tests on aspirated bone marrow cells

- Preparation of cell cytospins (for cytochemistry and immunocytochemistry)
- Flow cytometry ⎫ for analysis by monoclonal
- Fluorescence microscopy ⎬ antibodies of membrane and
⎭ cytoplasmic antigens on individual cells
- Cytogenetic examination, for example, Philadelphia chromosome in chronic granulocytic leukaemia
- DNA or RNA analysis, for example, detection of immunoglobulin or T cell receptor gene rearrangement
- Electron microscopy
- Semi-solid agar culture (for example, for diagnosis of myelodysplasia)
- Microbiological culture
- Deoxyuridine suppression test (for vitamin B_{12} and folate deficiency)

Bone marrow trephine biopsy

This is a more invasive procedure but it is essential for diagnosing those conditions that characteristically do not involve the bone marrow in a uniform manner (table). The morphology of individual cells is more difficult to characterise, but the overall architecture of the marrow is much better visualised (Fig 3). Trephine biopsy is essential for characterisation of marrow cellularity (whether aplastic or hyperplastic) and the degree of marrow fibrosis, and for detection of tumour infiltration by lymphoma and carcinoma. A trephine biopsy should always be obtained if the aspirate is unsuccessful; this can occur for technical reasons, if the marrow is fibrotic, or if particles of bone marrow have not been obtained and adequately spread following aspiration. In many cases, it is wise to obtain both types of specimen, because they provide complementary information.

153

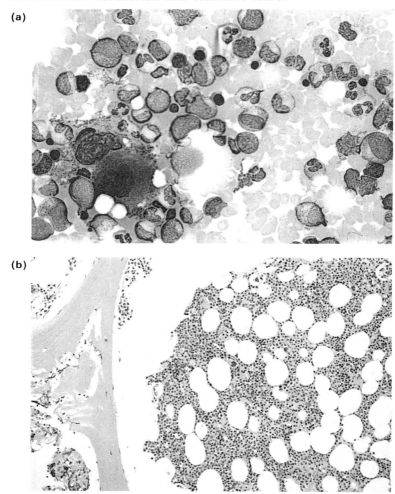

FIG 3 Normal bone marrow: the morphology of individual cells is much more easily seen in (a) the aspirate, whereas the overall architecture of the marrow is seen better in (b) the trephine biopsy

Indications

The indications for bone marrow aspiration and trephine biopsy have been shown in the table. When the marrow is to be used for marrow transplantation larger amounts of marrow (up to 500 ml)

154

are harvested under general anaesthesia from multiple puncture sites in the pelvis and sternum. Marrow for transplantation may be obtained from one of two alternatives: the patient's own bone marrow is harvested after primary chemotherapy, as part of a programme of intensive therapy (autologous transplantation); alternatively, it can be harvested from a volunteer, related or unrelated, HLA matching individual (allogeneic transplantation). It is usual to give a red cell transfusion at the time of bone marrow harvest and, in the case of a volunteer donor, this will usually be an autologous unit of blood obtained 1–2 weeks before the procedure.

Contraindications

The only major complication of bone marrow aspiration or trephine biopsy is haemorrhage at the site of the puncture. A full blood count and platelet count must always be obtained before the procedure, and a coagulation profile should be obtained if there is any reason to suspect an abnormality (for example, liver disease). Haemorrhage is much more common after trephine biopsy, which should not therefore be undertaken in patients having a severe coagulation defect without correction of the defect with appropriate therapy (for example, fresh frozen plasma or platelet transfusion).

Thrombocytopenia alone is not a contraindication, but platelet transfusion should precede trephine biopsy in patients with severe thrombocytopenia ($< 20 \times 10^9$/l) who either have evidence of bruising or bleeding, or have an abnormal coagulation profile.

Anaesthesia and sedation

Bone marrow aspiration is safely carried out in adults under local anaesthesia. As some adults will require serial examinations to monitor their response to therapy, it is important to make the procedure as comfortable as possible. Although the procedure may be performed in an outpatient setting, a day case admission is more appropriate especially if a trephine biopsy is also to be undertaken. Children may need general anaesthesia or heavy sedation.

Bone marrow trephine biopsy is best undertaken with the patient under sedation with generous local anaesthesia and as a day case admission. For adults, a short acting benzodiazepine (eg, intravenous midazolam up to 10 mg) given 30 minutes before the procedure is usually adequate. General anaesthesia is advised for children.

Equipment

- Clean trolley
- 2% plain lignocaine
- Syringes: 5 ml, 20 ml
- Needles: 19 gauge, 21 gauge
- Skin preparation (iodine or chlorhexidine)
- Sterile gloves
- Clean microscope slides and spreader
- Sterile dressing towels, swabs, and gauze
- Media/containers for specialised tests or culture
- Formalin container (for trephine biopsy)
- Bone marrow aspirate needle (with guard, either Salah or Klima)
- Bone marrow trephine needle (for example, Islam or Jamshidi–Swain)

Procedure

It is important to explain the procedure to the patient before starting. An assistant should be available.

Techniques

For aspiration

The posterior iliac crest is used in both adults and children. The medial aspect of the tibia, just below the tibial tubercle, should be used in infants below the age of 2. The body of the sternum may be used, for example, if the subject is obese and the iliac crest is inaccessible, or if the patient is unable to lie on his or her side. Aspiration may also be taken from the anterior iliac crest or from the spines of the lumbar vertebrae. For the posterior iliac crest approach, the patient is placed in the right or left lateral position with the back comfortably flexed.

Wearing sterile gloves, the area is cleaned with skin preparation and surrounded with sterile towels. The bony landmarks are identified. Aspiration may be performed from anywhere along the iliac crest, but it is usual to choose an area of the ilium lateral to the posterosuperior iliac crest (Fig 4). The skin, subcutaneous tissues, and (particularly) the periosteum are infiltrated with up to 10 ml 2% lignocaine. The aspiration needle with stylet and guard is assembled, the guard being essential for sternal puncture; it should be screwed 1–2 cm from the tip of the needle and adjusted so that, once the periosteum is reached, only a further 5 mm advancement is possible. However, for iliac crest and tibial procedures, the guard may be removed. The needle is held at right angles to the skin and advanced until the periosteum is reached. Maintaining the needle at right angles to the bone, it is then advanced firmly using a clockwise–counter-clockwise action to push it through the outer cortex of the bone. A sensation of decreased resistance is felt as the marrow cavity is entered.

The stylet is removed and a 10 ml syringe is attached to the needle. Sharp suction is applied and up to 0·5 ml marrow aspirated. Any larger volume will result in increasing contamination with peripheral blood, and marrow for ancillary tests should be taken into a separate syringe once slides have been prepared. If no marrow is aspirated, the needle is rotated or the stylet replaced, and the needle cautiously advanced or retracted. If marrow is still unobtainable, a different site along the iliac crest is attempted. Aspiration is sometimes successfully performed from the sternum in cases where iliac aspirate is unsuccessful.

For trephine biopsy

The patient is positioned and prepared as for posterior crest aspiration. Trephine biopsy should only be taken from the posterior iliac crest. The skin overlying the crest is incised with a scalpel blade or the site of entry of the aspirate needle may be used. The needle is assembled with the stylet locked in position and the handle grasped in the palm of the hand.

The needle is pushed through the subcutaneous tissues until it reaches the posterior crest. Maintaining the needle at right angles to the bone, it is advanced slowly and with firm pressure in an alternating clockwise–counter-clockwise motion until the outer cortex is pierced. The stylet is then removed and (for the Islam needle) the rounded head is placed on the needle. The needle is then advanced 2–3 cm in the direction of the anterior iliac crest. The needle should not be continuously rotated because this tends to distort and twist the core of the marrow within the needle. The

157

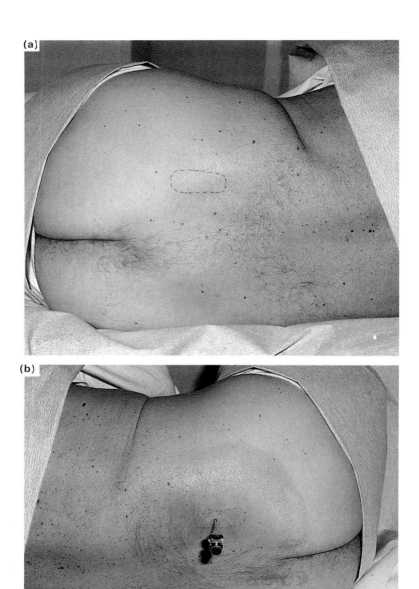

FIG 4 Both bone marrow aspiration and trephine biopsy are usually performed from the posterior iliac crest

needle is then withdrawn slightly (2–3 mm) and, with less pressure, advanced 2–3 mm further in a different direction. This will break the specimen at the distal cutting edge of the needle. The needle is then withdrawn slowly and the specimen is removed from the needle by introducing a probe through the distal cutting end.

After aspiration or trephine biopsy, firm pressure is applied to the site with a piece of gauze for three minutes or until bleeding has stopped.

The site is then covered with a plaster for 24 hours. Following trephine biopsy, the patient should be asked to lie on his or her back and thus apply weight over the biopsy site for 15–30 minutes.

The specimen

Aspirate

Smears must be made promptly before the specimen clots. This is a technique that requires practice, and badly prepared smears render the aspirate unacceptable. Single drops of aspirated marrow are placed onto slides about 1 cm from one end and most of the blood is sucked off with a fine Pasteur pipette applied to the edge of each drop. Alternatively, a few drops may be applied to a slide placed on a slope to allow the blood to drain away, leaving marrow fragments adhering to the slide. Films are then made, 3–5 cm in length, using a smooth edge glass spreader. The marrow fragments are dragged behind the spreader to leave a trail of cells. Satisfactory slides must include marrow particles as well as blood. Some haematologists prefer to place the sample into a full blood count specimen bottle containing dipotassium ethylenediamine tetra-acetic acid (K_2EDTA), and to prepare slides in the laboratory, using a Pasteur pipette. A paediatric tube should be used to avoid an excess of anticoagulant. A further modification is to place marrow fragments onto a slide and "squash" another slide on top to give a preparation in which the interior of the fragment may be viewed microscopically.

At least eight slides should be available for staining. Romanovsky (for example, May–Grünwald–Giemsa) and iron stains are carried out as a routine procedure, and further cytochemical stains may be required in certain circumstances (for example, to further characterise leukaemia cells). All slides should be fixed and unfixed slides should not be stored. Gloves must be worn while making marrow slides, and unfixed slides should not be handled without gloves.

Aspirated marrow for additional tests should only be taken after the slides have been made, and such material should be placed into appropriate containers. It is important to place such material (except, for example, when it is required for microbiological culture) into medium containing anticoagulant as soon as possible after aspiration.

Trephine

The specimen may be placed on a glass slide and an imprint made by gently rolling a fresh slide over the core. Such imprints ("roll preparations") may be stained with the aspirate slides. The trephine core is then placed into a histological fixative material for decalcification and sectioned and mounted in the histopathology laboratory.

Trephine cores are routinely stained by haematoxylin and eosin and by a silver technique for reticulin fibres. In some laboratories a plastic embedding technique is used. Additional stains and tests may be performed on the sliced trephine core – for example, immunocytochemistry or in situ hybridisation with nucleic acid probes. Some of these tests require the core to be placed in special media immediately after it is obtained, and the histopathology laboratory should be consulted before the biopsy if special tests are required.

Complications

Bone marrow aspiration and trephine biopsy performed by an experienced haematologist are safe procedures, and complications are extremely rare. However, the complications shown in the box have been reported.

Interpretation of results

The stained marrow aspirate films will be ready for examination 2–4 hours after obtaining the specimen. The slides are examined microscopically by an experienced haematologist who will assess the cellularity, proportion of various cell types, the appearance of

Complications

- Haemorrhage, especially after trephine biopsy: severe haemorrhage is only seen in patients with disordered coagulation (thrombocytopenia alone is not a contraindication). As mentioned above, it may be appropriate to conduct a clinical and laboratory assessment of haemostasis and to treat a haemostatic deficit before the procedure
- Bony perforation, especially when performing sternal aspiration. Failure to use the guard may lead to complete penetration of the bone with resultant fatal haemorrhage, pericardial tamponade, mediastinitis, or pneumomediastinum. Perforation is particularly likely in patients with brittle bones (for example, osteoporosis) or malignant infiltration of the bone marrow (for example, myeloma)
- Infection of the site of aspiration/biopsy; this is extremely rare if strict aseptic technique is used

the individual cells, and the presence of any abnormal cells. The results of specialised tests and examination of additional cytochemical stains will be available later. The trephine biopsy will usually be processed in the histopathology department and is available for sectioning and staining after decalcification, which may take several days. The stained sections should be examined microscopically by the histopathologist, the haematologist, or both, and it is useful to examine the trephine biopsy and aspirate films together.

Further reading

1 Hyun BH, Gulati GL, Ashton JK. Bone marrow examination: techniques and interpretation. *Hematol Oncol Clin North Am* 1988; **2**: 513–23.
2 Dacie JV, Lewis SM. Bone marrow biopsy. In *Practical Haematology*, 3rd Ed, London: Churchill Livingstone, 1991: 157–73.
3 Rothstein G. Origin and development of the blood and blood-forming tissues. In Lee GR, Bithell TC, Foerster J, Athens JW, Lakens JN, eds, *Wintrobe's Clinical Hematology*, 9th Ed. Philadelphia: Lea & Febiger, 1993: 41–78.

15 Aspiration and injection of joints

J M GUMPEL

Septic arthritis, diagnosed and treated early, need not lead to irreversible joint damage. Undiagnosed or inadequately treated joint sepsis often leads to irreversible joint damage, which is not amenable to joint replacement. Aspiration of potentially infected joints before use of antibiotics is therefore an important part of the repertoire of every hospital doctor. Although some cases of septic arthritis can be diagnosed circumstantially on the basis of positive cultures elsewhere, such as blood or wound swabs, only joint aspiration will give accurate information. Similarly, gout may be diagnosed clinically, but only the identification of intracellular uric acid crystals will give a definitive diagnosis.

In this age of disposable needles and syringes, therapeutic intra-articular and periarticular injections are practicable and mutually satisfying procedures in general practice.

This chapter cannot cover all the detail. If you would like to see the procedures carried out a visit to your friendly local rheumatologist in his or her clinic will get you started.

Visit your rheumatologist to see how it can be done

Indications and contraindications

The common indications for joint aspiration and for injection are shown in the box. Joints containing prostheses are the province of orthopaedic surgeons. Where sepsis is a possibility, corticosteroid injections are contraindicated until negative bacterial cultures have been obtained. Septic joints should be aspirated to "dryness" and aspirated daily until free from effusion. Acute haemarthroses should also be fully aspirated; in most other circumstances this is not necessary. Chronic indolent infection, especially with tuberculosis, is easily missed.

Avoid repeated injection of weight-bearing joints

Regularly repeated injections are thought to cause premature damage to the articular cartilage, and the need for repeated

---

Indications

Joint aspiration

Diagnostic
Undiagnosed acute effusion:
- ? septic
- ? crystal induced
- ? traumatic
- ? haemarthrosis

Therapeutic
- Tense acute effusion
- Interference with function
- Septic joint
- Haemarthrosis

Contraindications or special care
- Haemophilia
- Prosthetic joint

Joint injection

Diagnostic
- Arthrography – usually double contrast for meniscal tears
- Arthrography in investigation of calf pain or swelling
    ? ruptured knee capsule, *or*
    ? ruptured Baker's cyst

Therapeutic
- Persistent monoarthritis
- Enthesiopathy – for example, painful shoulder, tennis elbow
- Improve function – for example, in rheumatoid arthritis
- Peritendinitis

Contraindications or special care
- Infection, acute or chronic
- Prosthetic joint
- Repeated corticosteroid injections
- Athletic or overuse situations
- Achilles tendon

---

injection should be tempered by consideration of other factors – for example, poor muscle, joint instability, or damage requiring expert opinion. In athletes and other patients in whom overuse of joints has occurred, corticosteroid injections should not be considered an easy alternative to rest; in particular, the Achilles tendon is prone to rupture, particularly after inexpert injections.

Equipment

Chlorhexidine in spirit, or Hibiscrub and adequate washing facilities, sterile needles and syringes, and a no touch procedure are all the expert needs. For the less experienced, surgical drapes, gloves, and a sterile surface are important, and so is an adequate amount of lignocaine. Saline should be on the trolley: in the event of a "dry" tap, the saline can be used to check free flow into the joint and the washings can go for microbiological examination.

Equipment

- A rigorous aseptic no touch procedure
- Chlorhexidine in spirit
- Selection of syringes: 20, 10, 5, 2 ml
- Selection of needles: 19, 21, 23, 25 gauge
- Ampoules of local anaesthetic (without adrenaline)
- Ampoules of sterile saline
- Forceps (for jammed needles)

Optional
- Sterile cotton wool balls
- Sterile receiver or jug
- Sterile gloves
- Sterile drapes
- Sticky plasters
- Crêpe bandage

For injection
- Hydrocortisone *acetate* ampoules *or*
- Methylprednisolone acetate *or*
- Triamcinolone (hex)acetonide

Containers
- Sterile containers for microbiology, cytology (? + heparin), crystals (? + heparin)
- Lithium container for biochemistry, protein
- Fluoride container for synovial fluid glucose or blood glucose

---

Single dose ampoules are safest, unless you are the sole or first user of multidose phials. Do not use other people's ampoules. Hydrocortisone acetate is safe, cheap, and usually effective. Methylprednisolone acetate and triamcinolone (hex)acetonide may act for longer but are more likely to cause a post-injection flare and skin atrophy when injected close to the skin.

General procedure

Diagnostic aspiration or injection is much easier when appreciable swelling is present, as less precision is required in placing the needle. Before starting, carefully feel the bony margins of the joint space. Use the thumbnail to mark the joint space, and if in doubt move one bone so that you can feel its movement on one side of the joint. Check that all you need is easily available: choice of needles and syringes, local anaesthetic (or saline), requisite specimen containers, and, for large effusions, a jug or basin nearby. For aspiration followed by injection draw up the steroid beforehand and make sure the needles are not too tightly jammed on the syringes.

Get it all together before you start

Prepare the skin carefully with chlorhexidine in 5% spirit or surgical spirit – not Savlon. A rigorous no touch technique is for the experienced and for simple injections; sterile gloves, a sterile pack, and a generous area of prepared skin is for the less experienced. With experience it is rarely necessary to use local anaesthetic, and a subcutaneous bleb is usually sufficient. Local anaesthetic in the syringe is useful when difficulty in entering the joint is expected or to clear the needle and check that there is free and easy flow once the joint is entered.

Sterilise the skin over 5 inches (12·5 cm) before you start

In joint aspiration the needle size is important. For thick, purulent, or chronic effusions a white (19 gauge) needle is usually

165

needed; otherwise a green one (21 gauge) will suffice. For finger and toe joints use a blue (23 gauge) needle, which is usually used for injecting small quantities.

When effusions are purulent send specimens for microbiological examination and measurement of protein and glucose concentrations (in a small fluoride container), and a heparinised sample for cytology and crystal examination. Identifying crystals requires some experience, and at night it may be best to keep a sample refrigerated for re-examination next morning.

HIV-1 and acute arthritis

At the time of infection with HIV-1 or at the time of sero-conversion some patients with HIV develop an active synovitis which may affect one or several joints, often the knee. Some reports have suggested that many of these patients will have extensive psoriatic or psoriaform skin rash developing at this time. Where appropriate the doctor aspirating the knee should consider the need to use gloves and for special precautions, particularly in relation to the clinical situation of the patient as HIV-1 virus has been isolated and/or identified in synovial fluid in this clinical situation. Any of these procedures is very low risk.

Knee

The patient should be as comfortable as possible, lying down with sufficient pillows. The knee may be slightly flexed and muscles relaxed. Palpate the posterior edge of the patella medially or laterally and move it gently sideways to feel the femoral surfaces below. The patient should be sufficiently relaxed that the patella can be moved freely, otherwise aspiration is virtually impossible. Maintain a gentle conversation rather than grim silence. Insert the needle horizontally or slightly downwards into the joint in the gap between patella and femur (Fig 1); once behind the patella it must be within the joint. A slight resistance may often be felt as the needle goes through the synovial membrane. If no fluid can be aspirated check that the patient's quadriceps muscle is relaxed and that the needle is not blocked by injecting local anaesthetic. If this flows freely the needle is intra-articular. One last trick is to rotate the needle, as a synovial villous or fibrin body may be against the bevel.

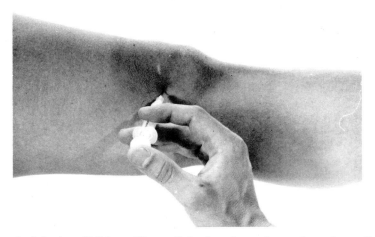

FIG 1   Injection of left knee. The needle has been inserted posterior to the patella. When there is no free fluid in the knee, more care needs to be taken to insert the needle in the space

Small effusions may sometimes be found in the medial or lateral pouches, and fluid will appear in the syringe as the needle is withdrawn very slowly with negative pressure. Once the correct position is found, rest the hand holding the syringe against the patient's leg. The usual dose is 50 mg hydrocortisone acetate, 40 mg methylprednisolone, or 20 mg triamcinolone (hex)acetonide. If injecting steroid do not completely aspirate the joint, so as to permit free diffusion of steroid around the cavity.

> **Always teach the patient a correct quadriceps muscle build-ing exercise programme**

Pre-patellar bursitis

Several bursae are present on the lower surface of the patella and patellar tendon. Although bursitis will usually respond to using a kneeling pad, some cases are sufficiently painful to warrant inject-ing 25 mg hydrocortisone acetate into the most tender area.

167

Ankle joint

With the foot slightly plantar flexed, palpate the joint line anteriorly between the tendons of extensor hallucis longus laterally and tibialis anterior medially just above the tip of the medial malleolus. Direct the needle slightly sideways, backwards, and upwards (Fig 2). Fluid may be aspirated if there is an effusion. Hydrocortisone acetate 25 mg is appropriate.

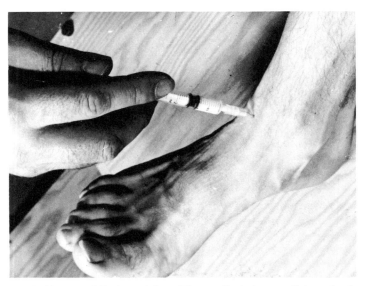

FIG 2 Ankles are difficult to inject. The needle is just medial to the lateral malleolus and just below the tibia

Shoulder (Fig 3)

The shoulder joint is most easily entered anteriorly: this route is used for aspiration, frozen shoulder, and synovitis. With the patient seated and his or her arm relaxed against the side of the chest, feel for the space between the head of the humerus and the glenoid cap, about 1 cm below the coracoid process. If in doubt, rotate the humerus by moving the extended hand outwards and feel the head moving under the fingers. Insert the needle into the space with a slight medial angle. It should enter the joint easily,

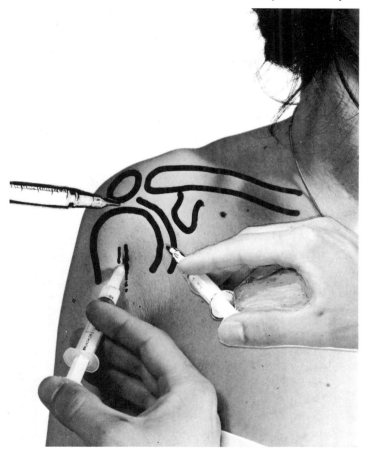

FIG 3   The routes for three different shoulder problems. The upper outer needle is in the supraspinatus bursa; the medial one is the shoulder joint "proper"; the lower one is almost parallel to the biceps tendon and the point is not in the tendon

almost to the length of a green (21 gauge) needle. The usual dose is 25–50 mg hydrocortisone acetate.

> **Carefully identify the correct site of pain. Refer to a textbook rather than rely on a patient's identification of the source of pain**

The lateral approach is used mainly for subacromial bursitis or the painful arc syndrome. Feel for the lateral tip of the acromium and insert the needle just below it in a medial direction with a slight downward slant until the tip reaches the humeral head. Gradually withdraw the needle with gentle pressure on the plunger: when the needle point is in the subacromial bursa a sudden drop in resistance will be felt. Injection will often reproduce the symptoms of the painful arc syndrome; if it does not, angle the needle in different directions until the pain is reproduced. Mixing local anaesthetic with the steroid is a useful diagnostic test, as the shoulder movements (or symptoms) should be improved after a few minutes. A second injection after a few days is often required.

Bicipital tendinitis is one cause of shoulder pain and is detected by finding tenderness over the tendon when the arm is externally rotated. Insert the needle almost parallel to the tendon – if it enters the tendon there will be resistance to the injection – then withdraw slightly and inject 25 mg hydrocortisone acetate into the tendon sheath and 25 mg direct into the shoulder joint, as part of the tendon is intra-articular.

Elbow (Fig 4)

Care is needed to differentiate between the possible sites of pain. Tennis and golfer's elbows are the common reasons for injection. The elbow is not an easy joint to inject, except in the presence of an effusion. The lateral approach is just proximal to the radial head, with the elbow flexed at 90°. Palpate the radial head while rotating the patient's hand, and locate the proximal end. Insert the needle between this and the lateral epicondyle at about 90° to the skin. The posterior approach may be used, again with the elbow at 90°, with the needle aimed between the olecranon process and the lateral epicondyle.

Tennis elbow

Carefully locate the site of maximal pain over the annular ligament of the radius and muscle attachments to it or to the lateral humeral epicondyle. Using a green or blue (21 or 23 gauge) needle, infiltrate (with considerable pressure) 25 mg hydrocortisone acetate and 1 ml local anaesthetic in and around the area of

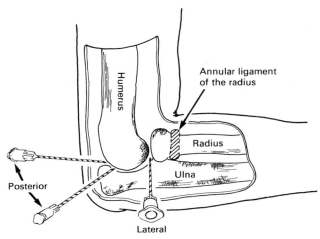

FIG 4   The posterior and lateral needles show routes into the elbow joint. If the lateral needle was 5 mm higher, it would be correct for lateral epicondylitis (tennis elbow); some patients with tennis elbow have pain mainly at the annular ligament

maximal tenderness, reinserting the needle down to bone in several areas without completely withdrawing it. After some five minutes check that the local tenderness has disappeared. A second injection is often needed after a few days.

> **Identify the most tender place, and check again before injection**

Golfer's elbow

Once again, carefully localise the maximal point of tenderness at the insertion of muscles into the medial epicondyle of the humerus and medial ligament, and inject as for tennis elbow. Remember to palpate and avoid the ulnar nerve in the groove below the medial epicondyle.

Wrist (Fig 5)

The easiest site for injecting the wrist is just distal to the ulnar head, on the dorsal surface of the wrist and slightly inside (to the

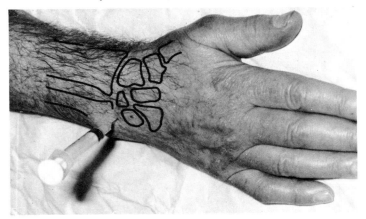

FIG 5   The needle is in the wrist joint just distal to the ulna, and "inside" or radial to the ulnar styloid

radial side). In theory several separate synovial cavities may exist, but in practice, particularly with persistent synovitis, usually all of these interconnect. Carefully palpate the space between the ulnar head and the lunate, and insert the needle at right angles to the skin between the extensor tendons to the ring and little fingers to a depth of about 1·0–1·5 cm. With careful palpation and marking, the needle will slip into a space between bones. The usual dose is 25 mg hydrocortisone acetate.

De Quervain's tenosynovitis

Tenosynovitis may occur in synovial sheaths surrounding the tendons of extensor pollicis longus and occasionally abductor pollicis longus as they pass through the extensor retinaculum on the dorsum of the wrist, and is usually apparent as a tender swelling along the tendons. Carefully palpate the swelling and insert the needle almost parallel to the skin, aiming it into the centre of the swelling. If the needle point is in the tendon injection will be difficult. Gradually withdraw the needle, with gentle pressure on the plunger, until free, easy flow occurs. The usual dose is 25 mg hydrocortisone acetate, but volume may be a problem: inject slowly, especially after 0·5 ml.

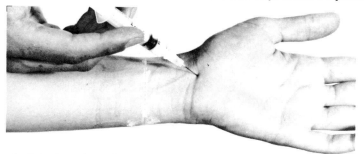

FIG 6   Injection of carpal tunnel: the needle is actually closer to the hook of the hamate than to the scaphoid tubercle (Fig 7). Some inject at the distal skin crease and some at the proximal crease

Hand (Fig 6)

Carpal tunnel

On the palmar surface of the hand the carpal tunnel is bridged by the flexor retinaculum (Fig 7), which runs between the hook of the hamate and the crest of the trapezium. These bony points are easily palpated at the level of the distal transverse skin crease. Insert the needle at right angles to the skin at this level, preferably closer to the hamate on the ulnar side, to avoid the median nerve, which is close to the trapezium, and superficial veins. The usual dose is 25 mg hydrocortisone acetate.

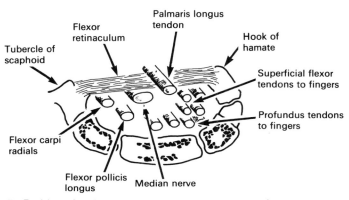

FIG 7   Position of various structures in a cross-section of the wrist at the carpal tunnel

173

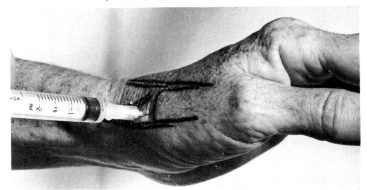

FIG 8   Injection of carpometacarpal joint. Above the joint, the tendon of extensor pollicis is outlined; below is that of abductor pollicis longus. In this space, the radial artery can usually be identified and avoided.

Palmar flexor tendons

Tenosynovitis of the finger flexor tendon sheaths may present as pain and difficulty on flexing the finger or as trigger finger. In the former case the tendon sheath feels thickened; in trigger finger a nodule on the tendon may be felt "popping" as the finger is flexed and extended. Carefully palpate the tendon in the palm with the fingers extended; insert the needle at the proximal skin crease of the finger, almost parallel to the course of the tendon and pointing towards the palm. Then proceed as for De Quervain's tenosynovitis.

First carpometacarpal joint of thumb (Fig 8)

Palpate the proximal margin of the first metacarpal bone in the anatomical snuffbox: flexion of the thumb into the palm of the hand will widen the joint space. Select a site between the long extensor and long abductor muscles; locate and avoid the radial artery. Insert the needle, pointing it at the base of the little finger, to a depth of about 1 cm. The usual dose is 25 mg hydrocortisone acetate.

174

16 Liver biopsy

JRF WALTERS
A PATON

Percutaneous needle biopsy of the liver is a simple bedside procedure that provides a core of tissue for laboratory investigation and so is valuable in many types of liver disease and systemic illness. Several different instruments are available, each with its own technique. The general principles apply to all, but our discussion of procedure is confined to the disposable Tru-Cut needle technique performed at the bedside. Guidance by ultrasonography in the radiology department is recommended for patients with mass lesions or small livers, and a "plugged biopsy" can be performed by the radiologist if there is a more than usual risk of bleeding. Liver biopsy may also be carried out at laparotomy and laparoscopy, and transvenously, but we do not propose to discuss these methods.

A blind procedure in an organ as vascular as the liver can be hazardous, so physicians should be well prepared and rehearsed. Practice with the appropriate instrument may be got in the necropsy room, but there is no substitute for learning by watching and copying someone who performs liver biopsies every week.

Contraindications

Can the patient understand the procedure and hold the breath for five seconds?

A violent cough or gasp when the needle is in position may tear the liver, with disastrous bleeding. A general anaesthetic is usually required in children.

175

Indications

- Confirmation of a clinical diagnosis of cirrhosis
- Investigation of chronic hepatitis and assessment of the effects of treatment
- Histological confirmation of primary and secondary tumours
- Investigation of "difficult" jaundice following demonstration of normal biliary ducts by ultrasonography or endoscopic retrograde cholangiopancreaticography
- Investigation of the effects of drugs, including alcohol, on the liver
- Occasionally in acute hepatitis and hepatomegaly, and when liver function tests give abnormal results that remain unexplained
- As an aid to diagnosing pyrexia of undetermined origin, granulomatous disease, and lymphomas

Is the patient likely to bleed excessively?

The prothrombin time is the best indication: if it is prolonged for more than three seconds and biopsy is considered to be essential then fresh frozen plasma should be given (one unit before, one during, and one after the biopsy); if it is over six seconds the procedure should not be carried out. When the prothrombin time is abnormal 10 mg vitamin K may be given parenterally for a few days. The platelet count is less important, but if it is below $50 \times 10^9/l$ (50 000/mm^3) care should be taken; platelet concentrations may be used.

Is the path to the liver normal?

Biopsy is best postponed when there is a skin or chest infection. Ascites causes the liver to float away from an advancing needle and when appreciable should be treated first.

Is biopsy likely to do more harm than good?

Patients with deep jaundice, especially from extrahepatic obstruction, where the bile ducts are dilated, risk biliary peritonitis as well as haemorrhage, and if cholangitis is present the infection may be spread. Biopsy should be undertaken only after appropriate treatment. Consider the possibility of a hydatid cyst, when anaphylaxis may result, or a vascular tumour including hepatoma, when angiography may be a better investigation.

Equipment

Check the trolley before you start and lay out the equipment, if possible away from the patient's bed. The items in the box should be present (Fig 1).

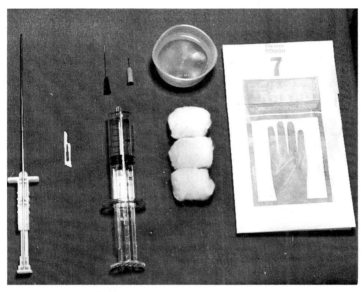

FIG 1   Equipment needed for biopsy (from top left): Tru-Cut needle, scalpel blade, needles and syringe of local anaesthetic, cotton wool balls and spirit, and disposable gloves

Equipment

- Plenty of cotton wool and gauze swabs
- Three or four sterile towels or drapes
- A small bowl of skin cleansing solution
- A 10 ml syringe for local anaesthetic
- A selection of hypodermic needles
- Sterile disposable plastic gloves
- A small scalpel blade
- Tru-Cut needle (test the movement of the trochar and cannula)

Before biopsy

Make sure the patient understands the procedure and has given informed consent.

Specimens of blood will have been sent to the laboratory for a full blood count, including platelets, prothrombin time, blood grouping and cross-matching, and standard liver function tests.

Ultrasonographic examination is routine and especially helpful when the liver is thought to be shrunken by cirrhosis or where bile ducts may be dilated by obstruction.

No restrictions need be placed on the patient's eating or drinking.

Procedure

The patient lies along the edge of the bed with the right arm behind the head, which is turned to the left. A pillow placed firmly along the left side of the body will keep it horizontal. Palpate the abdomen and percuss the liver in the mid-axillary line: remember that it is largely intrathoracic. Mark the rib space which is below the top of the liver dullness on full expiration (Fig 2). It may be helpful to mark the xiphisternum and liver edge as well.

Sedation is not usually necessary, but plenty of local anaesthetic is. Draw up 10 ml 1% lignocaine. Clean the skin and anaesthetise through a 25 gauge needle with a few drops of lignocaine in the appropriate space just above the rib. Then, using a 21 gauge needle, anaesthetise the deeper tissues with the patient breathing quietly, and advance slowly until a scratchy sensation or a gasp of pain indicates the sensitive tissues overlying the liver. Infiltrate this area with large amounts of anaesthetic. Remove the needle and, if you wish, measure the approximate distance to the surface of the liver on the biopsy needle.

Instruct the patient on how to take several deep breaths in and out and how to hold the breath in deep expiration for as long as possible. When you are satisfied with the manoeuvre nick the skin with the point of the scalpel blade, introduce the biopsy needle, and advance slowly with the patient breathing quietly. If you are not sure of the depth of the liver surface continue advancing cautiously until the needle begins to swing with respiration, then withdraw slightly until it stops swinging.

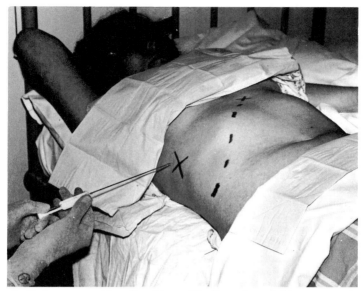

FIG 2   Patient prepared for a liver biopsy. The liver edge and skin puncture site are marked

Repeat the breathing instructions with the patient following you. As soon as the breath is held in expiration thrust the *closed* needle about an inch into the liver (Fig 3). Advance the inner

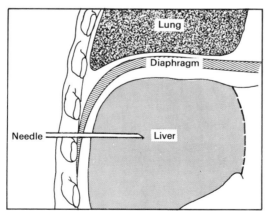

FIG 3   The anatomy around the liver biopsy needle tract

179

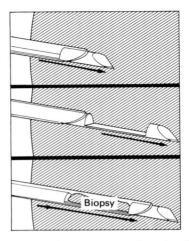

FIG 4   The sequence of movements used to take a liver biopsy

trocar, holding the outer cutting sheath still. Fix your right elbow against your side (to prevent the instinctive desire to withdraw the needle), advance the outer cutting sheath to cut the liver in the biopsy notch (Fig 4), and quickly withdraw the whole needle from the patient. With practice this sequence should take only a second or two. We prefer it to the one recommended by the manufacturer, because it ensures that the specimen is taken from within the liver rather than from under the capsule.

Cover the skin incision with a plaster and instruct the patient to lie on the right side for at least three hours. Pulse rate and blood pressure should be recorded frequently, and nurses instructed to report at once any alteration in condition or any complaint of pain.

The specimen (Fig 5)

Remove the biopsy specimen from the notch and divide it if specimens are needed for bacterial culture, biochemical examination, or electron microscopy in addition to histological examination. Place the histological specimen in 20 ml formol–saline on a piece of card to prevent fragmentation. Record the procedure in the notes, together with the texture of the biopsy specimen and its appearance to the naked eye: fat, pigmentation,

180

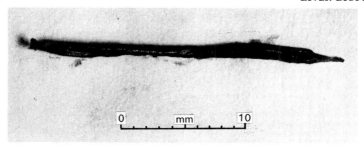

FIG 5   A large biopsy sample obtained using this technique

tumour, and cirrhosis can sometimes be recognised. Do not forget to note time of procedure, any instructions, and who to contact in the event of complications.

Complications

> ### Complications
> - No liver tissue obtained
> - Severe pain
> - Shock
> - Septicaemia
> - Rarer complications

No liver tissue is obtained

This occurs most commonly when the sequence of movements is incorrectly performed, the inner trocar being withdrawn when the outer sheath should have been advanced. Incorrect positioning (as in very fat people, when it may be difficult to outline liver dullness), inadequate expiration, and a small or mobile liver are other reasons. The experienced performer permits no more than two attempts at biopsy.

Severe pain

This may be caused by bleeding or leakage of bile. Pain in the shoulder tip and discomfort over the site of biopsy when the effect of the local anaesthetic wears off may require simple analgesia. Anything more than this should always be reported, and patient and nurses instructed accordingly. Biliary peritonitis is fortunately rare.

Shock

This is usually caused by rapid loss of blood from a large vessel or vascular tumour, less often by Gram-negative septicaemia. Bleeding may be more insidious, and blood transfusion should be started if there is unexplained tachycardia or hypotension, and fresh frozen plasma or platelets given if indicated.

Septicaemia

This may result from needling an infected bile duct or liver abscess and may be the first indication of infection.

Rarer complications

These include haemoptysis or pneumothorax owing to biopsy of the lung, and biliary or bacterial peritonitis owing to puncture of the gall bladder or colon respectively.

Anything more than slight pain or discomfort should be treated promptly and more serious complications must be considered an emergency. Consult a surgeon early. Though fortunately rare, death can occur from haemorrhage or biliary peritonitis, and delayed laparotomy contributes.

17 Kidney biopsy

P SHARPSTONE
JC KINGSWOOD

Patients with renal glomerular disease may present with similar clinical features and yet have conditions ranging from trivial to life threatening. Their prognosis and treatment depend on renal pathology, and histological examination of the kidney is often the only way to make the diagnosis.

Needle biopsy provides a sample of perhaps 20–30 of the 2000 000 glomeruli and so is unhelpful, and it may give misleading results in patchy conditions such as reflux nephropathy. It is most valuable in assessing and, in particular, indicating the prognosis of patients with diffuse glomerular disease.

Contraindications

Laceration of the kidney may cause haemorrhage, which could lead to nephrectomy. The risk is small but should always be kept in mind, and biopsy should be done only if the other kidney is adequate. The risk of doing a biopsy on a single kidney is acceptable in a renal graft. Contraindications are any haemorrhagic tendency including advanced uraemia. If biopsy is considered to be essential to management in a patient whose plasma creatinine is > 300 µmol/l, give desmopressin (DDAVP) 0·3 µg/kg in physiological saline by intravenous infusion over 60 minutes beforehand to minimise the risk of bleeding. The platelet count should be over $100 \times 10^9/l$ and the prothrombin time should give an international normalisation ratio of < 1·3. Control hypertension (blood pressure

Principal indications

Clinical syndrome	Indications for biopsy
Asymptomatic proteinuria	Protein excretion more than 1 g/24 h
	Red blood cells in urine
	Impaired renal function
Haematuria – macroscopic and microscopic	Imaging and cystoscopy exclude urological cause
	Proteinuria
	Impaired renal function
	Dysmorphic red blood cells and/or granular casts in urine
Acute nephritic syndrome	Persisting oliguria
Nephrotic syndrome	Adults: unless cause is apparent from extrarenal manifestations
	Children: only if haematuria also present, or if proteinuria persists after trial of corticosteroid
Acute renal failure	No obvious precipitating cause
	Obstruction of the renal tract excluded
Chronic renal failure	No major anatomical abnormality of kidneys
Renal allograft	To differentiate rejection, acute tubular necrosis, and cyclosporin A toxicity, and to diagnose recurrence of original disease

Equipment

- Tru-Cut disposable biopsy needles: 11·4 and 15 cm
- Exploring needle: 17 cm, 1·1 mm (19 gauge)
- Scalpel blade: no. 11
- Syringes: 10 and 2 ml
- Needles: 21 gauge (green) and 25 gauge (orange)
- 1% lignocaine: 10 ml
- Diazepam injection (Diazemuls) or midazolam: 10 mg/2 ml
- Skin disinfectant
- Sterile gloves, towels, and swabs
- Bath towel

higher than 160/95) before biopsy. Do not biopsy shrunken kidneys because they are difficult to locate, the histological findings are often non-specific, and in any case the result is unlikely to provide information of therapeutic relevance.

Before you start

Check the patient's blood pressure, blood urea and creatinine concentrations, haemoglobin, platelet count, and prothrombin time. Send blood to the laboratory for "group and save". Make sure that ultrasonography or an intravenous urogram has been done. Arrange a mutually convenient biopsy time for the operator and the radiologist who is to conduct ultrasonography. Check that the time is suitable for the histology technician to attend with a dissecting microscope. Explain the procedure to the patient and have him or her practice holding the breath in inspiration. Biopsy is unsafe if the patient cannot cooperate. Obtain an informed consent in writing.

Procedure

Renal biopsy is potentially hazardous, and the inexperienced should do it only under skilled supervision. Premedication with intravenous diazepam makes the procedure less unpleasant for the patient; general anaesthesia is required only for infants or young children. A firm surface is needed, and to "fix" the kidneys roll up a towel (about 10 cm in diameter) and put it under the patient's abdomen between the rib cage and the pelvis. Place the patient prone with his or her head turned away (most patients do not want to watch), the arms abducted, and the forearms beside the head.

Ultrasonography is used to locate the kidney (Fig 1). The site of choice is the edge of the lower pole of the left kidney. This avoids major renal vessels and is likely to contain more cortex than medulla. Mark it on the skin and note the depth of the kidney there (Fig 2).

Wear sterile gloves and stand at the left side of the patient. Prepare the skin and locally anaesthetise the skin and subcutaneous tissues; then use an exploring needle to find the kidney. Insert it into the lumbar muscles and then advance it 5 mm at a time until a definite swing with respiration shows that the point is within the

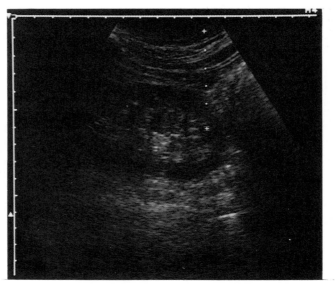

FIG 1   Ultrasonic image of kidney showing track biopsy needle to lower pole

kidney. Ask the patient to hold his or her breath in inspiration each time you move the needle and to breathe out and in after each advance. Do not restrict movement of the needle while the patient is breathing: handle it only while the patient is holding his or her breath. After locating the kidney inject local anaesthetic along the track, especially around the capsule, while withdrawing the needle.

The 11·4 cm Tru-Cut needle is suitable for most patients, but use the 15 cm one for larger patients (Fig 3). Make a nick in the skin with the point of a scalpel blade and then advance the biopsy needle, with the cannula closed over the obturator, stepwise as with the explosing needle. A large arc of swing usually shows that the kidney has been located, but beware the patient who uses the chest more than the diaphragm when asked to breathe deeply. When the swing is small it is easy to penetrate the full thickness of the kidney, and the specimen obtained will comprise only fat or blood clot. In these patients correct location of the point of the needle depends on feeling the resistance of the capsule and the "give" on penetrating it. The disposable needle is sharp and the

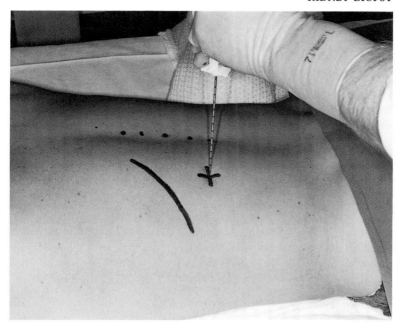

FIG 2   Site of biopsy in relation to lower border of twelfth rib and lumbar spinous processes

change in resistance slight; so, for sensitive control, hold it low down by the shaft rather than by its handle. A small jerk with each respiratory movement means that the tip of the needle is just scraping the capsule and should be advanced a little further. If the needle moves only at the extreme of inspiration it is probably being struck by the lower pole and should be reinserted higher up.

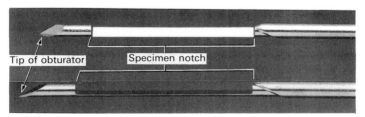

FIG 3   The "business end" of a Tru-Cut needle

When you are satisfied that the tip is *just* within the kidney ask the patient to hold his or her breath in inspiration. Then tap the obturator handle in, push the cannula smartly down the length of its travel to cut the specimen, keeping the obturator handle firmly fixed with the other hand, and finally withdraw the needle with the cannula closed over the obturator. The last three manoeuvres must be made while the patient is holding his or her breath, so practise them on a ripe pear first.

Troubleshooting

A successful biopsy produces a strip of kidney up to 20 mm long. The various histological techniques require the specimen to be divided up into at least three portions, so examine each with a dissecting microscope and make sure that all contain glomeruli. If there is any doubt about their adequacy obtain another specimen rather than risk having to repeat the whole performance later on when you receive the histological report reading "medulla only".

The specimen (Fig 4)

Immunofluorescent microscopy is carried out on fresh tissue, whereas routine, immunoperoxidase, and electron microscopy require appropriate fixatives. Consult the histopathology laboratory about its requirements or, preferably, arrange for a technician to collect the specimen.

Make sure that details are included on the request form which are necessary for a helpful interpretation of the histological investigation, such as the patient's age, blood pressure, renal function, amount of proteinuria, multisystem disease, and drug history.

Aftercare and complications

The patient should remain in bed for 24 hours and have his or her pulse and blood pressure checked every hour for four hours and then every four hours. Advise the patient to avoid strenuous exercise for the next week.

The most important complication is haemorrhage, which could be perirenal, causing loin pain and sometimes a palpable mass, as well as the signs of blood loss; additionally, it could be intrapelvic,

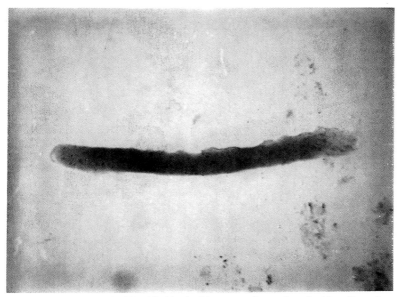

FIG 4   Glomeruli can be identified in the biopsy specimen viewed with a dissecting microscope

causing persisting heavy haematuria and sometimes clot retention. More minor haematuria is common and usually settles quickly. Continuing haemorrhage should be treated by blood transfusion and sedation and, if necessary, selective embolisation after arteriography to locate the source. Exploration of the kidney is only rarely required.

Interpretation of results

Even the most experienced and skilled renal histopathologist cannot give all the answers, even in diffuse glomerular disease; remember the sampling error in focal lesions.

18 Intravenous urography

B CRAMER
G DE LACEY
C RECORD
L WILKINSON

Intravenous urography (IVU) provides anatomical information about the urinary tract. During the last decade ultrasonography has developed as the first line investigation in preference to the IVU in several well defined situations. In particular ultrasonography is recommended as the first imaging technique when assessing renal size and outline, investigating suspected hydronephrosis, and for evaluating a suspected mass lesion. Renal function is more accurately assessed using radiolabelled isotope studies than on the IVU.

Indications

1 Renal colic or pain related to the upper urinary tract. In some departments, a plain radiograph and ultrasonography are preferred
2 Haematuria when ultrasonic examination of the kidneys is reported as normal
3 In some cases of suspected trauma to the upper renal tract
4 Infection:
  (a) suspected tuberculosis of the urinary tract
  (b) in women an IVU is indicated only if it is a complicated infection, e.g. infection associated with loin pain, haematuria, or raised serum creatinine[1]
  (c) in infants and children urography is not considered to be a useful first line investigation[2,3]

Indications

The availability of diagnostic ultrasonography has affected the selection and sequence of imaging techniques in most situations. Indeed there are now few circumstances in which the IVU is the undisputed first line investigation. Bearing this in mind, and recognising that the precise choice of technique should be tailored to the individual patient, indications for IVU are those shown in the box.

Contraindications

There are no absolute contraindications to IVU, but those in the box are relative contraindications.

Contraindications

- Known sensitivity to contrast media, asthma, or a strong history of allergy[4]
- *Cardiac disease*: the risk factor is increased fivefold in patients with heart failure; this risk increases with the severity of the heart disease[4]
- *Renal failure*: transient rises in serum creatinine occur after intravascular contrast medium,[5] and acute-on-chronic renal failure may be precipitated, particularly with high doses of contrast, in patients with diabetes mellitus, and in patients who are dehydrated[6]
- Hypertensive crises may be precipitated in patients with *phaeochromocytoma*; these patients should be covered with α- and β-adrenergic blockade[4]
- *Myeloma*: contrast media may cause precipitation of Bence Jones protein. Large doses of contrast medium should be avoided and patients should be well hydrated[4]
- *Neonates*: the kidneys may not be visualised within 48 hours of birth despite normal renal function[4]
- The IVU should be avoided in women of childbearing age in whom pregnancy is a possibility, unless there is an overwhelming clinical indication[6]
- *Pregnant women*: irradiation to the fetus should be avoided whenever possible. If unavoidable, the examination should consist of a preliminary film, and a full length erect film 25–30 min after administration of contrast medium[6]

The need for intravenous urography should be assessed in all these patients, and alternative imaging methods strongly considered. If intravenous urography is essential, then the patient should be well hydrated both before and after the procedure, and a low osmolar contrast medium should be used.[6] Patients with a history of severe asthma, or previous severe contrast reaction, should receive prophylactic prednisolone (50 mg orally, at 13, 7, and 1 hour before the examination).[7]

Contrast media

The risk of non-fatal reactions is reduced by a factor of three- to sixfold when low osmolar agents are used,[7] and more patients experience minor effects such as nausea and urticaria when high osmolar agents are used (table).[5] Low osmolar contrast media should be used in children and in all patients with the risk factors listed above. However, it has been argued that as the low osmolar contrast media are up to six times as expensive as high osmolar contrast media, the latter should be used for all other patients.

Age and indication	Dose	Iodine equivalent (mg/ml)	Osmolality
Adults			
Routine	50 ml	420	High
High risk	70 ml	300	Low
Renal failure	2 ml/kg body weight	300	Low
Children (based on body weight)			
Up to 12 kg	1·5 ml/kg body weight		Low
12–40 kg	18 ml + 1 ml/kg for each kg above 12 kg	300	Low

Preparation

The patient should remain ambulant before the examination to minimise the presence of bowel gas. Laxatives are not generally considered useful.[9]

Patients should not be dehydrated as this increases the risk of precipitating renal failure.[5]

192

Equipment

- Contrast medium; both high and low osmolar agents should be available
- 19 gauge butterfly needle (smaller gauge for children)
- Quill
- Antiseptic swabs
- Tape
- Tourniquet
- Compression band
- Vomit bowl
- Emergency drug box

Suggested drugs to be kept[8]

In the emergency box
  Chlorpheniramine maleate
  Promethazine
  Hydrocortisone succinate
  Salbutamol inhaler
  Salbutamol nebuliser
  Ephedrine
  Physiological saline
  Gelofusine

For use by the crash team
  Methoxamine
  Dobutamine
  Dopamine
  Adrenaline 1:10 000
  Adrenaline 1:1000

It is advisable to avoid a large meal before the examination as some patients experience nausea following the injection of contrast medium.

A history of possible contraindications should be elicited. When appropriate, a low osmolar contrast medium should be used and steroid prophylaxis given where appropriate.

Normal procedure[5]

The patient should empty the bladder immediately before the

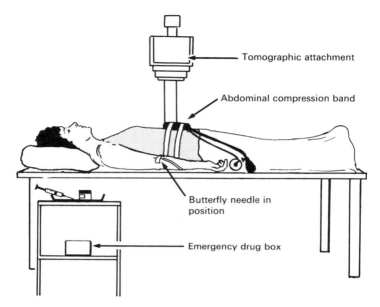

Equipment required for an intravenous urogram

procedure, and a control abdominal radiograph is taken. The patient lies supine on the table, and the contrast medium is injected rapidly via a median antecubital vein.

Suggested radiograph sequence

- Immediate post-injection radiograph, restricted to the renal area, to show the outlines of the kidneys
- Five minute radiograph, restricted to the renal area, to show the calyceal system
- Fifteen minute radiograph to show the entire renal tract

Modifications

1 Abdominal compression may be applied after the five minute radiograph if the calyceal system is not well distended. In this case, an additional ten minute radiograph, restricted to the renal

area, is obtained, with tomography if necessary. Contraindications to compression include:

(a) renal colic;
(b) recent trauma;
(c) recent abdominal surgery;
(d) a large abdominal mass.

2 Simple linear tomography may be required to delineate poorly visualised renal outlines and collecting systems.

3 In a patient with urinary tract obstruction, further radiographs may be needed. The interval at which delayed radiographs are obtained will depend on the severity of the obstruction. For instance, if there is an obvious mid-ureteric calculus on the plain radiograph and delay in excretion on (say) the five minute radiograph, then no further radiographs are indicated. In some other circumstances delayed radiographs will be necessary to delineate the level and/or cause of the obstruction.

4 In children and infants, the rate of injection should be slow. A fizzy drink may be given to produce a gas filled stomach, which acts as a window through which to view the kidneys.

5 In renal failure, a low osmolality contrast medium is used, and the dose increased.[4] The patient must be well hydrated.

Complications and aftercare

Intravenous contrast media can cause drug reactions, which may be life threatening or even fatal. All doctors directing an IVU should be familiar with the treatment of possible reactions.

● Patients with unpleasant symptoms such as flushing, nausea, metallic taste, shivering, and sneezing should be reassured.

● Most minor reactions such as urticaria, rhinitis, and conjunctivitis may also be treated conservatively. However, an antihistamine, such as oral or intravenous chlorpheniramine maleate 10 mg, is appropriate.[4]

● Bronchospasm may occur, especially in asthmatic individuals, and may be quite severe. Oxygen, nebulised salbutamol, and intravenous hydrocortisone succinate 100 mg should be given.[4]

● Acute anaphylaxis (manifest by urticaria, bronchospasm, and glottic and angioneurotic oedema) may lead to circulatory collapse and pulmonary oedema. Oxygen, hydrocortisone, and

195

antihistamines should be given as above. Subcutaneous adrenaline (0·5 ml 1:1000 solution) should also be given in severe cases.[4]

- Vasovagal reactions and cardiac arrest can also occur. Treatment should be administered by experienced medical staff, with anaesthetic support if necessary, according to the nature of the episode.

Interpretation of results

- The control radiograph will show renal tract calcification whether in the renal parenchyma, the collecting system, the ureters or the bladder. It may also be used to assess the residual urine volume following micturition.
- The immediate radiograph shows the nephrogram, and is used to delineate renal size, shape, and position.
- The pelvicalyceal systems and ureters should be inspected for dilatation (local or generalised), persistent narrowing, distortion, deviation, and delayed or incomplete filling.
- The bladder outline is inspected for diverticula, trabeculation, and an elevated bladder base caused by prostatic hypertrophy. Filling defects may be more obvious on a post-micturition film. However, it is emphasised that the IVU is a crude and inaccurate method of evaluating the bladder for small papillomas and this is best carried out by cytoscopy.

References

1 De Lange EE, Jones B. Unnecessary intravenous urography in young women with recurrent urinary tract infections. *Clin Radiol* 1983; **34:** 551–3.
2 Whitaker RH, Sherwood T. Another look at diagnostic pathways in children with urinary tract infections: *BMJ* 1984; **288:** 839–41.
3 Sherwood T, Whitaker RH. Initial screening of children with urinary tract infections: is plain film radiography and ultrasonography enough? *BMJ* 1984; **288:** 827.
4 Grainger R. Intravascular contrast media. In Grainger R, Allison D, eds, *Diagnostic Radiology*. Edinburgh: Churchill Livingstone, 1991.
5 Dawson P. Intravenous urography revisited. *Br J Urol* 1990; **66:** 561–7.
6 Whitehouse G. The urinary tract. In Whitehouse GH, Worthington BS, eds, *Techniques in Diagnostic Imaging*. Oxford: Blackwell Scientific, 1990: 281–94.
7 Ansell G. Adverse reactions profile: Intravascular iodinated radiocontrast media. *Prescribers' Journal* 1993: **33**(2): 82–88.

8 Guidelines for the management of reaction to intravenous contrast media. *Royal College of Radiologists Recommendations.* FCR/1/93 January 1993.
9 Bailey S, Tyrrell P, Hale M. A trial to assess the effectiveness of bowel preparation prior to intravenous urography. *Clin Radiol* 1991; **44:** 335–7.

19 Administering cytotoxic chemotherapy

SE BEACH
J MIDDLETON
J LUKEN
PPB JAMES
CJ WILLIAMS

Cytotoxic drugs have a narrow therapeutic index, with significant potential for harm. They are most often used for palliative rather than curative purposes, and their use is best restricted to those experienced in cancer chemotherapy. Anyone administering chemotherapy should be fully familiar with all aspects of each of the cytotoxic drugs used.

Indications

For palliative treatment the simplest effective treatment should be used and stopped at the first sign of tumour progression or unacceptable side effects. When treatment is potentially curative, every attempt should be made to reduce toxicity while maintaining intensive drug doses.

Considerations before preparing chemotherapy

- Blood count – low platelets and/or neutrophils will necessitate dose reduction or delay. Most chemotherapy schedules include advice on how to do this.
- Organ function and toxicity – organ-specific toxicities are not uncommon; for example anthracyclines, such as doxorubicin, can cause or worsen cardiac failure. Hepatic and renal dysfunction may contraindicate use of certain cytotoxics, or necessitate dose reductions (Box A). A knowledge of organ-specific toxicities is therefore a prerequisite for using any cytotoxic drug.

Box A   Cytotoxic drugs and organ failure

Dosages of certain drugs must be reduced or omitted in:

- Renal impairment – methotrexate, cisplatin, carboplatin, bleomycin, streptozocin

- Hepatic impairment – anthracyclines (doxorubicin, daunorubicin, epirubicin, idarubicin), vinca alkaloids (vincristine, vinblastine, vindesine)

- Cardiac failure – anthracyclines, mitozantrone

- Infection – usually a reason for postponing treatment.
- Drug dosage – usually calculated according to the patient's surface area, which is obtained from a nomogram using the patient's height and weight.
- Route and rate of drug administration.
- The extravasation potential of the drug (see below).

Preparation of injectable cytotoxic drugs

Ideally the drugs should be drawn up by staff in a properly equipped pharmacy. Current guidelines include:

- Preparation should be on a named patient basis.
- Use protective clothing, that is, gloves, safety glasses, surgical face mask, a disposable water repellent gown.
- A safety cabinet or isolator should be used if possible, otherwise a separate designated well ventilated area will suffice.
- Use Luer-Lok syringes, and air inlet devices when preparing drugs in rubber topped vials.
- Excess air should be expelled into the sheath of a clean needle or back into the vial.

    Always check the compatibility of the drug, diluents and intravenous solutions.

Administration

- Ensure the patient is comfortable, a task made easier by explaining the procedure to the patient, and answering any questions he or she may have. Explanation will reduce anxiety and will in turn help reduce problems such as nausea and vomiting which are partly mediated through conditioning. Patients should

199

receive a clear explanation of likely side effects such as hair loss, nausea and vomiting, low blood counts, etc.

- All patients receiving chemotherapy should be given a contact phone number which they may use, at any time of the day or night, to get advice and help.
- With aseptic technique, an indwelling cannula or butterfly needle is inserted into a vein on the forearm or back of hand. (The antecubital fossa may be used for bolus injections should this be the site of the largest vein; infusions should be administered through a more peripheral vein.) Ensure that the tape used to keep the intravenous line stable does not obscure the site of entry of the needle.

Vesicants

These drugs can cause severe irritation if extravasated:

- Actinomycin
- Doxorubicin
- Daunorubicin
- Epirubicin
- Idarubicin
- Etoposide
- Mitomycin

- Mustine
- Vincristine
- Vinblastine
- Vindesine
- Dacarbazine
- Mithramycin (plicamycin)

- Check the cannula is functioning and the vein is patent by flushing with at least 5 ml sodium chloride 0·9% BP. If there is any suggestion of extravasation the needle must be resited.
- Inject the drug in the manner recommended by the data sheet. If using vesicant drugs these should be injected before other drugs and into a fast running drip.
- Watch the patient and the vein throughout. Ask him or her to report any discomfort or abnormal sensations. If there is any sign of swelling or pain when a vesicant is being injected, *stop immediately*. Follow the recommended policy in your unit for dealing with extravasation (Box B).
- After injection, flush with at least 5 ml sodium chloride 0·9% BP to prevent leakage. Remove intravenous device and apply a sterile dressing.

Intrathecal injection

Warning

Intrathecal chemotherapy should not be prepared or given at the same time as intravenous chemotherapy

---

For all intents and purposes, only methotrexate and cytarabine are given by the intrathecal route. The drugs and any diluents must be preservative free. If a CSF sample is required for analysis it should be taken before injecting the drugs.

Troubleshooting

- Extravasation (Box B).
- Local reactions – redness and irritation sometimes develop along the vein being injected as a local reaction to the drug, especially when small veins are used. This may be reduced by further dilution of the drug.
- Pain on injection – some drugs (especially dacarbazine, mustine, and vinblastine) can cause muscular and venous pain on administration. This pain is felt along the vein and not just at the site of the cannula, so is different from that caused by extravasation. Further dilution or injection into a fast running drip often helps.

Box B Measures to be taken following extravasation

- Stop injection, leave needle in place
- Aspirate as much drug as possible
- Remove needle
- Give hydrocortisone 100 mg as about eight subcutaneous injections around the circumference of the extravasation site*
- Apply ice or a cold pack
- Reapply ice or cold pack for 15 minutes every 6 h
- If ulceration develops, obtain plastic surgical advice
- Complete any reporting documents required by local policy

*The use of steroids is controversial and subject to local policy

---

Aftercare and complications

Nausea and vomiting

Many cytotoxics can cause severe emesis. It is essential to achieve the best possible antiemetic control from the outset. This will be dictated by unit policy, taking into account the degree of emesis usually seen with the cytotoxics being used. Do not wait for the patient to start vomiting before commencing antiemetics.

Myelosuppression

Patients *must* be instructed to contact your unit at *any* time they become unwell, febrile, or have a possible infection. They must be seen immediately if neutropenia is a possibility; sepsis during

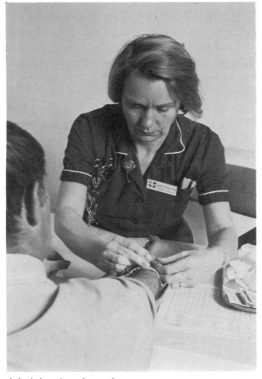

Administering chemotherapy

neutropenia may be fatal within hours. Patients with a neutropenic fever should be admitted to hospital for intravenous broad spectrum antibiotics.

Stomatitis

Patients should be advised about oral hygiene and should contact you if they develop severe ulceration or pain.

Coloured urine

Patients should be warned that their urine may become (harmlessly) coloured for some hours after the administration of certain drugs.

Cytotoxic drugs

These cause a wide variety of side effects and those administering such treatment should have a thorough knowledge of these and their management.

A final word

The administration and management of intravenous cytotoxic drugs require specialised knowledge. If you are in any doubt about their use please ask someone experienced in cancer chemotherapy because these drugs can be lethal if misused.

Part III
Minor surgical procedures for hospital and primary care

20 Suturing

H ELLIS

Suturing neatly and quickly is one of the important arts that should be acquired, as soon as possible, by house surgeons or casualty officers. Even if they do not propose to pursue a career in surgery they will find this of value if their future lies in many other branches of medicine – general practice, anaesthesia, or even morbid anatomy.

Most suturing experience in the early days is connected with lacerations, and it is this aspect that will be dealt with here. The advice given also applies to closure of the skin in the operative wounds encountered in main theatre or after minor surgery in the accident and emergency or outpatient department.

Contraindications

Small, superficial cuts will heal well if cleaned with a suitable detergent disinfectant, such as chlorhexidine, and covered with an adhesive dressing. This applies particularly to minor scalp lacerations within the hairline. Small children may not tolerate closure of a clean cut by sutures under local anaesthetic. Rather than submitting them to a general anaesthetic (and the subsequent trauma of having the sutures removed), their clean cuts can be disinfected, dried with spirit, and the edges apposed with Steristrips (Fig 1).

If there is extensive skin loss, so that the wound can be apposed only under considerable tension, the surgeon should call in a more senior colleague. Such wounds may need closure by mobilising a

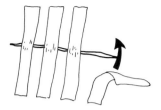

FIG 1   A small, clean wound closed with Steristrips

local flap of skin or, more commonly, by means of a skin graft – not to be attempted by the unsupervised trainee.

Severely contused or heavily contaminated wounds, particularly when there has been a delay of six hours or more before surgery, should not be treated by primary suture because of the considerable risk of wound infection and breakdown. The wound should be cleaned and excised (as described below) and dressed with dry gauze. In the absence of infection, delayed primary suture can then be performed on the fifth day, with excellent prospects for satisfactory healing. A similar technique should be used in dealing with high velocity injuries – for example, gunshot wounds – in which, again, primary suture of the wound is likely to be followed by infection and wound breakdown. The only exceptions to this rule are contused or high velocity wounds of the head and neck. Here the magnificent blood supply of these tissues enables the surgeon to carry out primary suture with minimal risk of necrosis or infection.

Instruments and equipment

A very good rule, which cannot be learned too early, is to check all instruments and equipment carefully before performing any operative procedure, no matter how minor this might be. This will obviate the embarrassment to the operator and the discomfort to the patient of such experiences as inserting a sigmoidoscope before making sure that the obturator can be removed or that the light will turn on.

Even for the relatively minor procedure of suturing a laceration there is quite an armamentarium to look over. The instruments required are shown in the box.

Instruments

- Scalpel handle size 3 with scalpel blades 10 and 15 (or a disposable scalpel)
- Stitch scissors
- Three to six fine artery forceps (depending on the extent of the wound)
- Needle holder
- Toothed dissecting forceps
- Fine catgut for ligating blood vessels (3/0)
- Fine nylon (3/0) attached to a straight or curved cutting needle, depending on the operator's choice

---

For local anaesthesia, 1% lignocaine with adrenaline, a disposable syringe, and disposable fine needles will be required.

Warning

Do not use adrenaline containing solutions near end arteries (eg, fingers, toes)

For skin preparation either iodine *or* a detergent disinfectant solution such as chlorhexidine is needed.

In addition, the operator will require sterile disposable gloves, sterile dressings, sufficient sterile towels to drape the wound, Micropore to secure the dressings, and, if the laceration affects the arm, a triangular bandage or a collar and cuff to use as a sling.

Before you start

A simple explanation of what you are proposing to do should be given to the patient (or, in the case of a small child, to the parents). If the wound is extensive, contaminated to any degree, or caused by a perforation (for example, by a garden fork), consider the risk of clostridial infection. Check on the patient's tetanus immunisation and, if necessary, give a "booster" dose of tetanus toxoid. In all but perfectly clean lacerated wounds, start penicillin prophylaxis by intramuscular injection (use erythromycin in patients who are sensitive to penicillin).

Most patients can have their lacerations sutured by means of simple local anaesthetic infiltration. A particularly nervous patient may require a preliminary intravenous injection of diazepam in a dose of between 5 and 20 mg. A smaller dose is indicated in elderly subjects.

Procedure

Procedure
- Clean and sterilise around the wound
- Infiltrate local anaesthetic
- Excise any dead or necrotic tissue
- Ensure that serious injury is not present
- Suture the wound closed
- Ensure haemostasis achieved
- Apply dry dressing

In dealing with a lacerated wound the surgeon's aims are:

- To remove dead, devitalised tissue and any foreign contaminated material to reduce to a minimum the risk of wound infection
- To stop bleeding
- To approximate the skin edges (and, if necessary, the deep tissues) neatly and without undue tension to ensure as cosmetically favourable a result as possible.

A wide area of skin around the wound is carefully cleaned and then sterilised – for example, if the laceration involves the hand, the skin, from the forearm down to the fingers, is prepared. If the skin is dirty it may need repeated scrubbing with soap and water. If hairy skin is involved a wide area around the wound is shaved and for this a disposable razor is particularly useful. Lacerations of the scalp should be widely cleared of hair; it is surprising how often an extension of the laceration or a second wound is discovered when blood stained, matted hair is cleared away.

Once the skin is clean, a wide area around the wound is disinfected with iodine or chlorhexidine and the area draped with sterile towels.

Local anaesthesia (Fig 2) is achieved by infiltration with 1%

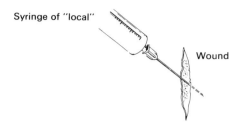

Syringe of "local"

Wound

FIG 2   Infiltration of anaesthetic into a wound

lignocaine with adrenaline. If the initial injection is made within the lips of the wound, and if a fine needle is used, infiltration, even of the relatively extensive wounds, can be carried out almost painlessly.

Once the wound has become anaesthetised (and this is within seconds of infiltration) the lips of the wound are opened and the interior carefully explored. If there is an obvious spurting artery this is picked up at once with artery forceps. A large "spurter" may need to be tied off with 3/0 catgut. Small blood vessels can be treated by picking up with artery forceps, leaving the forceps on for a minute or two, and then twisting the forceps round and round before removing them. This torsion technique is very effective and saves burying a good deal of catgut in the wound. Scalp lacerations can bleed quite profusely. Here a useful technique is for the assistant to press firmly with the fingers on either side of the laceration down onto the scalp (Fig 3). Once the surgeon has

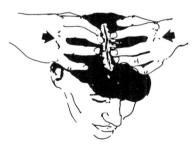

FIG 3   Pressure on the underlying skull on either side of a scalp laceration controls the bleeding

sutured the wound, the bleeding will cease simply as a result of the compression effect of the stitches.

A clean incised laceration needs no excision. In the case of contused wounds or crush injuries, the edges of the wound require excision back to healthy bleeding tissues. Usually the skin edges themselves require only minimal trimming with the scalpel (and this is particularly so in the highly vascular tissues of the scalp, face, and neck). However, the deeper tissues, particularly fat, should be excised more widely and the surgeon should ensure that only healthy, vascular bleeding tissue remains in the depths of the wound. Any foreign material (glass, fragments of clothing, road debris) must be carefully sought after and removed (Fig 4).

It is the casualty officer or the house surgeon's duty to make sure what looks like a relatively minor wound does not conceal a more serious injury. In the case of a scalp laceration check that there is no underlying communication with a fracture. If the wound is over a joint make sure that the joint itself has not been opened; of course, lacerations of the wrist need careful preoperative and operative assessment to exclude injury to tendons, nerves, or major vessels. In any of these eventualities, send for help!

If the laceration is deep, the deep tissues may need to be apposed with a few interrupted catgut sutures, and this applies also to the divided aponeurosis in a scalp laceration. Closure of the skin itself should be carried out, in most instances, by means of simple interrupted fine nylon sutures placed 2 or 3 mm from the skin edges (Fig 5). Sutures placed further from the skin edges simply result in ugly "cross-hatched" scars. The knots should be positioned away from the skin edge and tied at just sufficient tension to

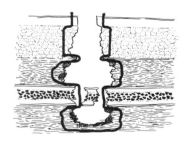

FIG 4   Remove all dead and foreign material

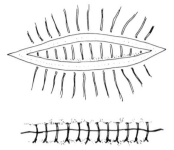

FIG 5   Simple sutures tied away from the edge of the wound

appose the lips of the wound to each other (Fig 6). Tying the knots tightly simply strangulates the underlying tissues, whereas if the sutures are slack, underlying fat tends to push out through the wound edges with a resultant ugly scar.

Mattress sutures should be used only if the surgeon finds difficulty in apposing the skin edges (Fig 7). Unlike the simple sutures, the knots here should be tied at the wound edge itself.

The only other "fancy" suture that may be required is in the

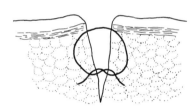

FIG 6   Fine catgut to appose the deep layers

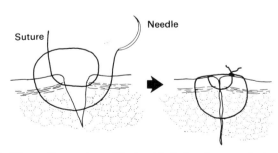

FIG 7   The mattress suture. The knot is tied at the wound edge

213

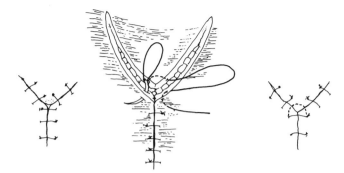

FIG 8   How to suture a Y or V laceration

case of a triangular or Y shaped wound (Fig 8). The apex of the triangle is transfixed with a subcuticular stitch (as shown in the diagram) to prevent a gap at this point.

After ensuring that haemostasis has been achieved and that the wound has been neatly brought together, a dry dressing is applied and held in place with Micropore.

Suture of drains and drainage tubes

The house officer may be called upon to suture in place a latex rubber or plastic drain or drainage tube (for example, a suprapubic catheter or a chest drain).

A simple nylon stitch, loosely tied, is all that is needed in the case of a drain. Cut the ends of the suture long, so that there is no confusion between the stitch which holds the drain and the wound stitches. Also place a large safety pin through the drain just above the skin surface; the stitch prevents the drain from falling out and the safety pin stops it from falling in (Fig 9a), an accident that is not unknown.

When stitching in a tube drain, the stitch should not pass through the tube itself, this may cause leakage and is to be avoided especially with an underwater tube drain in the chest. A stitch is placed and tied alongside the tube; the ends of the suture are left long and are then employed to plait firmly around the tube and then tied to form a "Roman sandal" effect (Fig 9b). To remove the tube, all that is necessary is to cut the suture at its base.

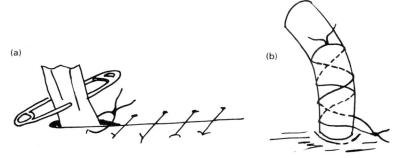

FIG 9   (a) A corrugated drain secured by a nylon stitch. The ends are left long for easy identification. A large safety pin prevents the drain disappearing into the wound. (b) A tube drain secured by a "Roman sandal" knot

Aftercare

The patient should be provided with suitable oral analgesics and told to report at any time if the wound should ooze or become uncomfortable.

Sutures on the scalp, face, and neck heal with great rapidity and these can be removed in three or four days. The less time they remain, the neater the scar. When there is tension or when movement of the part may pull on the wound – for example, on the hand – the sutures should remain for 10–14 days – better a few days too long than to have the wound gape and require a secondary suture.

21 Surgery for lumps, bumps, and skin lesions

TH BROWN
NA SCOTT

Removal of skin lesions and subcutaneous lumps is common in general surgery and dermatology. In addition, many general practitioners are increasingly expected to perform these procedures. Despite the apparently trivial nature of this surgery, problems can arise if basic surgical principles are not adhered to. The surgeon needs to consider the points in the box before embarking on removal of any skin or subcutaneous lesion.

- What are the indications for excision?
- What are the disadvantages and risks to the patient?
- Is there adequate equipment available?
- Which local anaesthetic and how much is appropriate?
- Which skin suture and when should they be removed?
- Is histology required?

Indications

Skin lesions and subcutaneous lumps are removed for a number of reasons.

Indications

Diagnosis
Cosmesis
Discomfort
Sepsis

Diagnosis

The precise nature of the skin lesion may require histological examination. Pigmented naevi can be a source of considerable anxiety to a patient. However, a positive clinical diagnosis should be made without resorting to surgical removal of every pigmented lesion – if in doubt ask for a senior opinion.

Cosmesis

Patients complain that a subcutaneous lump or skin lesion is unsightly.

Discomfort

A subcutaneous lump may be painful or might "catch" when combing hair, or rub on clothing.

Sepsis

Recurrent infections can occur with sebaceous cysts.

Cautions to consider

When discussing the pros and cons of removing a skin lesion the following should be considered.

Scarring

All surgical incisions leave a scar, the dimensions and prominence of which vary according to the size of the lesion, the site of excision, and the surgical techniques used. Keloid formation can be a problem over the chest wall and sternum. Scars from wounds on the back can "spread" to occupy an area similar to that of the excised skin.

Each patient should be warned about scarring and, in some circumstances, they will decline excision when this has been discussed. Large lesions on the face should not be tackled by the inexperienced, but may require referral to a plastic surgeon.

Size and depth of lesion

Some subcutaneous lumps can be too large for easy removal under local anaesthetic. The amount of local anaesthetic agent used needs to be considered carefully because too much can produce toxicity.

217

Similarly, the depth of an apparently subcutaneous lump can be significantly underestimated. Lumps in the neck can feel very accessible for local anaesthetic removal to the unwary; such misjudgements rapidly become evident to the surgeon and the patient as the attempted excision proceeds.

Other factors

Patients on anticoagulants may be at risk of haematoma formation. A record of therapeutic anticoagulation is not a contraindication to minor outpatient surgery.

Equipment and local anaesthetic

Setting

Minor surgical procedures, like all invasive techniques, require strict attention to asepsis. A suitable clinical area or operating room should be available with good lighting for these procedures. For most excisions it is best if the patient can lie down on a couch or operating table. This both helps exposure of the operative site and stops the occasional patient fainting. Suitable "easy listening" music (e.g. Radio 2's Gloria Hunniford programme) may help defuse the clinical atmosphere for the patient.

Equipment

Minor operating set should contain the items shown in the box.

Nos 3 and 4 scalpel handle
Four curved and four straight mosquitoes
One toothed and one non-toothed dissecting forceps
One Volkman's spoon
One suture scissors and one dissecting scissors
One needle holder
Gallipot and swabs
3/0 absorbable ties and 3/0 monofilament suture
Syringe and needles for infiltration anaesthetic

Skin preparation solution
Formalin jar
(Bipolar diathermy – doesn't need plate on patient)

Local anaesthetic solutions

The two principal infiltration anaesthetic agents used for minor surgery are lignocaine (0·5, 1, and 2% solutions) and bupivacaine (0.25 and 0.5% solutions). Both are available as either a "plain" injection or in combination with 1:200 000 adrenaline solution. The principal difference between the two agents lies in the speed of onset of action (lignocaine is faster than bupivacaine) and their duration of action (bupivacaine lasts longer than lignocaine). The addition of adrenaline to the local anaesthetic prolongs the duration of action, increases the amount of anaesthetic that can be used, and facilitates surgery by reducing bleeding. However, adrenaline-containing local anaesthetics must not be used near end arteries, for example, fingers and toes.

For successful and safe local anaesthesia the following principles should be followed:

- Avoid intravascular injection of the local anaesthetic (aspirate before injection).
- Be aware of the maximum permitted dose of local anaesthetic (lignocaine plain 200 mg, with adrenaline 500 mg for adult).
- Allow time for the local anaesthetic to work before starting surgery (infiltrate operative site before scrubbing up).

The procedure

Skin preparation (Fig 1)

The skin over the lesion should be shaved to provide a clear view and prevent hair falling into the wound. The skin is cleaned for a generous distance around the wound and the operative field towelled off.

Anaesthetic infiltration

A fine needle is used to raise a weal of anaesthetic at two or three points around the lesion. A larger needle (Fig 2) is then introduced and the operative field infiltrated with local anaesthetic. The patient should be warned that he or she will feel the initial needle prick and that the local anaesthetic will sting as it is injected. (This stinging can be reduced by warming the ampoule of local anaesthetic.)

Time should now be allowed for the local anaesthetic to take

219

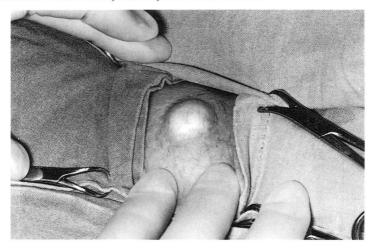

FIG 1   Skin preparation: the area is adequately shaved

effect before surgery is started. Patients should be told that they will be aware of pressure and movement during surgery but no pain. They should be asked to alert the surgeon to any pain so that more local anaesthetic can be infiltrated if necessary.

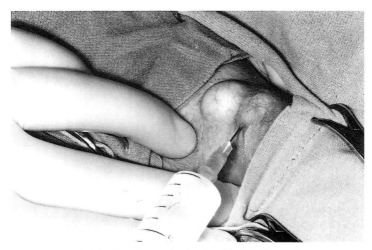

FIG 2   Local anaesthetic: the skin is infiltrated

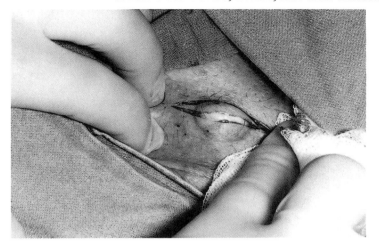

FIG 3   Skin incisions: an elliptical incision is often used

Incision

An elliptical incision is usually made around the lesion or over the subcutaneous lump to be removed (Fig 3). If a potentially malignant skin lesion is being excised, the surgeon needs to decide whether the aim of the procedure is just diagnosis or whether it is adequate clearance and local control of the possible malignancy. If the procedure is an excision biopsy for diagnosis a formal margin of clearance is not necessary. Confirmation of malignancy will then mandate a second excision of the biopsy site with formal margins. By contrast, excision of a skin lesion for local control of a malignant lesion entails making formal *measured* margins from the edge of the lesion.

Dissection (Fig 4)

Sebaceous cysts and lipomas are dissected out by developing tissue planes with a curved mosquito or curved scissors. Haemostasis can be obtained by crushing small vessels, ligation, or bipolar diathermy. Brisk bleeding from scalp wounds is best dealt with by suturing the skin closed and, if necessary, applying a pressure dressing.

221

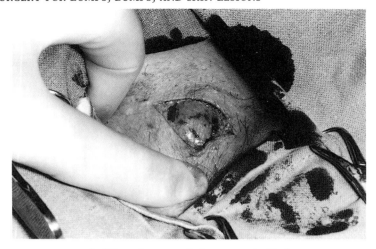

FIG 4   Dissection: wound after removal of lesion

Skin closure

For the large majority of skin lesions and subcutaneous lump removals, skin closure can easily be obtained with a series of interrupted 3/0 monofilament sutures (Fig 5). Finer suture

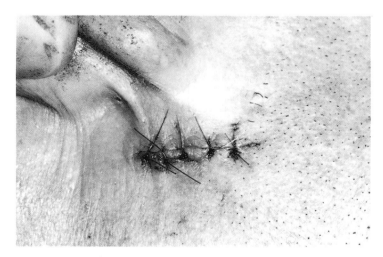

FIG 5   Skin closure: interrupted, monofilament sutures

material can be considered on the face. Steristrips and subcuticular polypropylene (Prolene) closure can also be used.

Wound dressing and care

Facial wounds are not usually dressed, and wounds elsewhere can be covered by Airstrip or Micropore dressings. Plastic spray dressings can be useful for scalp wounds.

Normally wounds should be occluded while bathing or showering. Timing of suture removal depends on the site and the individual surgeon.

Complications

Complications
Bleeding
Wound infection
Wound separation

Bleeding

This is usually controlled by pressure. If it persists it may be necessary to consider reopening the wound to remove clot and control the bleeding point.

Wound infection

This is rare after minor skin surgery, and is usually dealt with by removing a suture and allowing the wound to drain.

Wound separation

This can be associated with wound infection. Re-suturing can be considered, but allowing healing by secondary intention can also produce a satisfactory result.

Histological investigations

All skin lesions removed for diagnostic purposes need to be sent for histological examination. In addition, any "doubtful lesion" should also be submitted to pathological scrutiny. Each specimen must be clearly labelled before the patient leaves the operating room. The request card requires clinical details of the lesion and the suspected clinical diagnosis. Finally, all histological results must be seen and signed by the clinician who performed the excision. Such a system prevents unexpected histological findings being filed away without appropriate action being taken.

Summary

Surgical excision of skin lesions and subcutaneous lumps is part of general surgery, dermatology, and general practice. The indications for each excision must be carefully considered along with the possibility of adverse scarring.

Success depends on good patient explanation, good infiltration anaesthetic technique, and adequate facilities and equipment. After the procedure the patient must be clear about wound care, suture removal, and who to see about any wound problems. Finally, great care must be taken in sending specimens for histological examination and then ensuring that each histological result is seen and acted upon by the relevant clinician.

Further reading

Dando P. *Medico-legal aspects of minor surgery*. London: Medical Defence Union, 1991.

---

22 Drains and sutures and their removal

TH BROWN
S HUGHES

Drains and their use

Drains are used to remove fluid or air from a body cavity or wound. They are often placed at the end of an operation to ensure adequate removal of fluid from the operative site (that is, the peritoneal cavity or neck), but can also be used for the percutaneous removal of pus or blood after insertion under local anaesthetic using ultrasonography or computed tomography guidance.

In this way a drain provides a mechanical means of removing material which could be harmful to the patient or detrimental to recovery after surgery. Pus can be drained from an abscess, air from a pneumothorax, blood from the pelvis after extensive surgery, or urine from an obstructed renal system.

Types of drain (see box)

Comparison of suction and non-suction drains		
	Suction	*Non-suction*
Placement	Stab wound	Incision
Fluid removal	Active	Passive
Infection risk	Closed system	Open system
	Minimal risk	More risk
Exit site	Clean	Fluid discharge
	Easy to manage	May get skin irritation

225

Non-suction drain

Non-suction drains provide a route of least resistance from the peritoneal cavity to the skin. They can be corrugated, smooth, or tubular and allow a means of escape for the blood or pus. Once placed they require a skin suture to hold them in place. There is no suction associated with this drain so the exit of fluid is passive. Their major disadvantage is that they can allow bacteria to track up the drain and into the patient.

Suction drain (Fig 1)

To provide an active means of extracting fluid, suction has been added to drainage systems. A tubular drain is used (most commonly size 10, 14 or 18 French gauge); the last 5–10 cm contain multiple side holes. The drain is introduced through a stab incision and held in place with a skin suture. The external end attaches to the suction device. The initial devices used high pressure, but this can lead to omentum, bowel, or other tissue being caught in the holes of the drain and damaged during its removal. This risk has been overcome by the use of low suction drainage devices. In these devices the suction pressure is obtained by a collapsible receptacle which can be compressed and attached to the tubing.

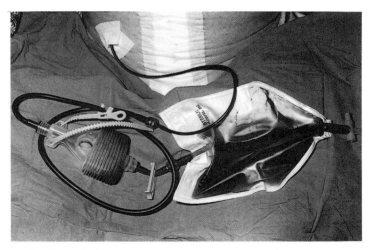

FIG 1 Suction drain in situ; note the closed system, concertina suction drain, and drainable collecting bag

Special purpose drains

T tube drainage

The short limbs of a T tube (Fig 2a) are placed in the gastrointestinal tract, with the long arm brought out through the skin. This allows controlled drainage from the gastrointestinal tract (Fig 2b). A T tube is usually placed in the common bile duct after supraduodenal exploration for the removal of stones. After 7–10 days a cholangiogram is obtained down the T tube to show adequate flow into the duodenum and no retained stones. If the cholangiogram is satisfactory the T tube can be removed. A T tube can also be used in the jejunum for decompression and tube feeding should this be required.

Removal of drains

Non-suction drains

These drains can be shortened before they are removed by cutting the retaining skin suture, pulling the drain out 4–5 cm and placing a safety pin near the skin to prevent retraction into the peritoneal cavity. Removal of such drains requires a sterile trolley, suture cutter, and scissors (if shortening of the drain is being undertaken). Having cut the holding suture the drain is pulled firmly but steadily until removed. Care is taken to ensure no damage to the drain, and minimal discomfort to the patient.

Suction drains

Before removal of these drains, suction is disconnected to prevent the sucking of tissue from the peritoneal cavity into the drain, and their subsequent removal with the drain. The retaining suture is divided and a pair of forceps placed on the tubing. The forceps are pulled to extract the drain, and pressure applied to the drainage site to prevent bleeding.

Skin closure

Wounds in the skin heal, unless there is continued irritation by a discharge, a foreign body, infection, or deliberate interference. Healing will occur by primary or secondary intention, and the aim of skin closure is to achieve the former. The technique used to

(a)

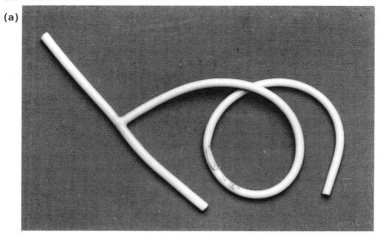

(b)

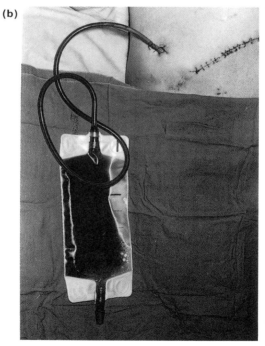

FIG 2   T tube: (a) T tube showing long limb and shorter T section; (b) T tube in situ with collecting bag

228

achieve skin closure will not heal the wound but will approximate the skin edges to ensure the minimum distance across which to achieve healing. The ideal skin closure is when the two edges lie parallel, with no in-turning of the edges, no infection, no foreign body, no distracting tension, and no ischaemic tension in the sutured tissue. This should lead to a clean, tidy wound with no visible suture marks.

Removal of skin suture

Timing

The timing of the removal of skin sutures or clips depends on the position of the wound, the type of surgery that has been done, the direction of the wound (transverse, midline, skin crease, etc) and the presence of complications. The timing of this removal is indicated in the box.

Timing of removal of sutures	
Site	Approximate timing (days) of removal
Head and neck (e.g. thyroidectomy)	3–4
Laparoscopy	3–5
Hernia, appendicectomy	5–7
Laparotomy, perineal wounds, thoracotomy	7–14
Back	14

Technique

Simple suture

The equipment needed for this includes a basic dressing trolley and a stitch cutter (Fig 3a). Having explained to the patient what will happen, the trolley is prepared and the wound is cleaned. A piece of gauze is used to receive the removed sutures. The knot of each suture is firmly grasped with a pair of forceps and gently elevated to pull the stitch away from the skin (Fig 3b). The stitch

(a)

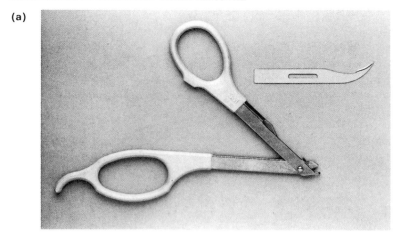

(b)

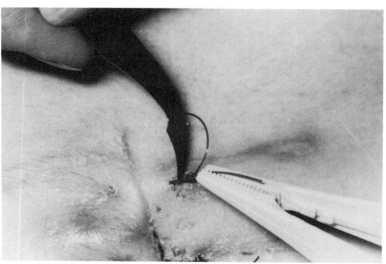

FIG 3 Suture removal: (a) staple remover and suture cutter; (b) cutting suture –
suture held with forceps and divided with cutter

cutter is used to cut the suture next to the skin, and the knot is gently pulled to remove the suture.

Subcuticular suture with beads

A subcuticular suture with a bead at each end can also be removed using the same basic equipment. One of the beads is held by the pair of forceps and retracted from the skin. The suture is cut close to the skin and removed by gentle traction on the opposite end of the suture.

(a)

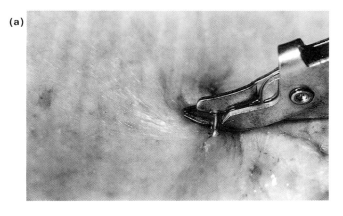

(b)

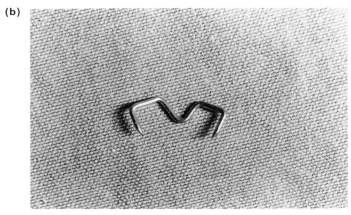

FIG 4   Staple removal: (a) staple remover placed through staple; (b) extracted staple – bending the staple into an "M" shape extracts it from the skin

Skin clips

These can be removed using a similar dressing trolley and a pair of clip or staple removers (Fig 3a). The preparation and cleaning of the wound are the same as for the suture removal. The staple remover is then inserted with the double arm under the staple and the single arm over it (Fig 4a). As the handles are squeezed together the ends of the staples are distracted, thus extracting them from the skin and folding the staple into an "M" shape (Fig 4b).

23 Vaginal examination and taking a smear

E FORSYTHE

A vaginal examination includes inspection of the external genitalia, a bimanual digital examination, and an internal examination of the vagina using a speculum. It should always be preceded by an abdominal examination. If the examination is done with sensitivity on the part of the doctor and with the full cooperation of the patient it can help with the diagnosis of not only physical problems but also psychological and sexual ones.

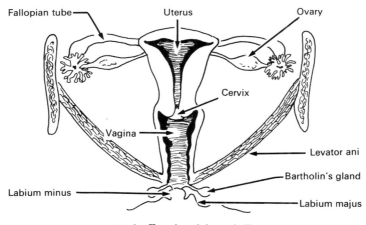

FIG 1   Female pelvic genitalia

Indications

- A screening procedure including the taking of a smear
- Part of a general gynaecological examination to investigate gynae-cological signs and symptoms
- Obstetric management
- Investigation of a genitourinary problem
- In the family planning consultation for excluding gynaecological disease, before fitting an intrauterine contraceptive device or a diaphragm, or in the investigation and treatment of a psycho-sexual problem
- The investigation of wider clinical problems including lower abdominal pain, endocrinological abnormalities, or lower limb oedema

Contraindications

Possibly the procedure is contraindicated for the virgin of any age (Fig 2); but if the patient is relaxed and there is good communication between the doctor and the patient examination may be possible with one finger and the use of a very small speculum.

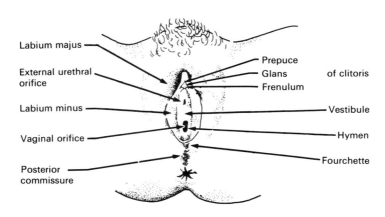

FIG 2   The vulva of a virgin

Equipment

- An examination room screened from sight and, if possible, from sound
- A standard bench type couch with a waterproof covering and disposable paper coverings
- An efficient adjustable light
- Disposable plastic gloves
- K-Y or other lubricating jelly
- A variety of sizes of bivalve specula (Fig 3) including one suitable for the examination of a virgin
- A Sims' speculum (Fig 3)
- Swabs, forceps for holding a sponge, and long Spencer–Wells forceps
- A clean towel or sheet for covering the patient's abdomen and thighs
- Tampons and sanitary pads
- For taking a smear: glass slides, a pencil for writing the patient's name, a choice of spatulas, fixative, and a slide holder for transport
- For taking swabs: sterile swabs and transport media for bacteria and viruses as supplied by the laboratory
- The correct forms for sending with the specimens
- A microscope for the immediate diagnosis of *Trichomonas* sp.

Note — all instruments should be autoclaved

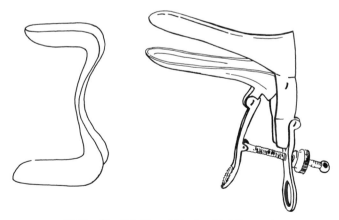

FIG 3   Sims' (left) and bivalve (right) specula

Before you start

The laboratory should be alerted if results are required urgently. The investigation of chlamydiae and herpes viruses needs rapid transport to the laboratory – certainly within 24 hours.

Check that the patient has emptied her bladder, unless she is being examined for prolapse or stress incontinence. Arrange for the collection of a midstream specimen of urine, if necessary.

Before taking a smear check that the patient has not had sexual intercourse in the previous 24 hours and has not inserted a diaphragm.

Procedure

A male doctor usually prefers to have a chaperone present. It is important that the doctor talks to the patient during the examination, explains what he is doing, and remains aware of the patient's feelings.

Latex gloves must be worn on both hands and routine precautions taken to avoid contamination with body fluids.

The dorsal position is the most commonly used (Fig 4b). The patient lies on her back with her knees flexed and her hips flexed and abducted. Her abdomen and thighs should be covered so that she feels less exposed. Raising the head of the couch makes the patient more comfortable and helps her to relax. She will be able to see what the doctor is doing and may be less apprehensive. However, she may prefer to be in the position in which she has been examined previously.

The left lateral position is useful for the woman with reduced mobility of her hips and the very embarrassed patient (Fig 4a). It gives good exposure of the anus, perineum, and the posterior parts of the vulva, and is useful for examining, with the Sims' speculum, a prolapse in an obese patient.

It is helpful to make physical contact with the patient while you explain the procedure to her – for example, if she is in the dorsal position your left hand could be rested against her right knee. If she shows distress at any time during the examination you must discover whether it is because of pain, fear, her embarrassment, your embarrassment, or your clumsiness. The examination follows

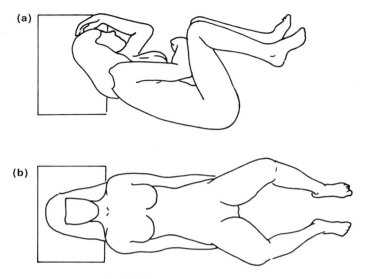

FIG 4   (a) Left lateral position; (b) dorsal position

a sequence from external genitalia, vagina, cervix, uterus, adnexae, and pouch of Douglas.

External inspection

Notice if there is a smell – for example, the bad smell of a retained tampon. Inspect the urethral opening for a discharge, urethritis, or a caruncle. Ask the patient to cough and observe if there is any leakage of urine and to push down to look for any prolapse. Note also any vaginal discharge, the state of the skin, the presence of an intact hymen, ulceration, tumour, warts, or herpes. Take swabs if necessary.

Internal inspection

This should be done before bimanual digital examination if a smear is to be taken. The size of the speculum used will depend on the patient's menstrual, sexual, and obstetric history. If the internal inspection of a virgin is to be attempted choose a very small speculum. Warm the speculum in warm water and check the

237

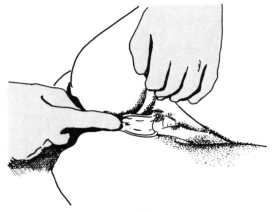

FIG 5   Insertion of Sims' speculum

temperature against your gloved hand before use. Water or a small amount of lubricant can be used to ease its passage.

While standing at the right of the patient hold the speculum in the right hand and with the left hand gently separate the labia minora. The speculum can be introduced with the blades vertical or at an angle of 45° from the vertical (Fig 6). As the blades enter the vagina rotate them until they are horizontal, exerting gentle pressure against the posterior wall of the vagina. Observing the direction of the vagina, push the speculum upwards and backwards until the blades can be opened to expose the cervix (Fig 7). Difficulty in exposing the cervix may result from using too large or too short a speculum, the speculum being too far anterior or posterior, or to vaginismus. Note the size, shape, and appearance of the cervix. Is there ulceration, erosion, a polyp, tear, or discharge?

Taking a smear

Have the marked slide and fixative ready. The cells to be examined must come from the squamocolumnar junction, which may be inside the cervical canal (Fig 8). Good exposure of the cervix is vital. Insert the forked end of a wooden or plastic spatula into the cervical canal and rotate it through 360° (Fig 9). Exert enough pressure to sample the cells, but do not press hard enough to cause bleeding. Spread the material thinly on the slide. Spray

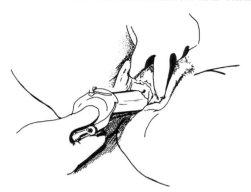

FIG 6   Introducing the bivalve speculum

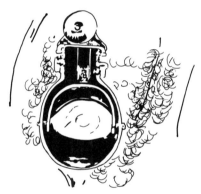

FIG 7   Exposure of cervix

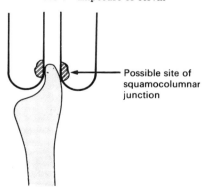

Possible site of
squamocolumnar
junction

FIG 8   Spatula sampling squamocolumnar junction

239

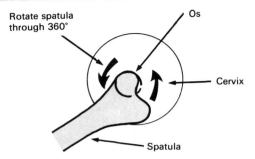

FIG 9 Use of spatula for taking smear

immediately with fixative or immerse in fixative. After 10–15 minutes drain off surplus fixative and put the slide in a transporter.

A cytobrush is useful if the squamocolumnar junction is within the canal.

Taking a swab

For ulcers use a dry sterile swab and swab firmly from the base of the lesion. For chlamydiae swab from around the cervix and into the endocervical canal. For vaginal discharge take a swab from high up in the posterior fornix. Break the end of the swab off and place it in the appropriate medium. Check the method of culture used for chlamydiae with the local laboratory and arrange suitable refrigeration and transport.

The blades of the speculum must open slightly during withdrawal, so that the cervix is not caught between the blades because this is uncomfortable for the patient. The walls of the vagina can best be observed during removal of the speculum. Any discharge or surplus lubricant left on the vulva should be gently wiped away with a swab. If necessary the patient should be given a tampon or pad.

Bimanual digital examination

This can be done before internal inspection if you are not taking a smear. Insert the well lubricated index finger of the right hand (some doctors use two fingers but this is more uncomfortable and seldom necessary) into the vagina while separating the labia minora with the left. The left hand is then placed on the abdomen

240

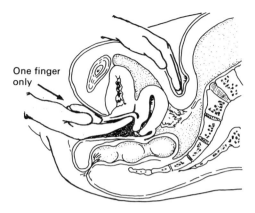

FIG 10   Position of hands during bimanual pelvic examination

below the umbilicus and moved slowly downwards. The hand on the abdomen is more effective for feeling the pelvic organs than the finger(s) in the vagina (Fig 10). The finger in the anterior fornix pushes the cervix as far backwards as possible. The uterus can then be brought forwards and palpated between the right finger and the left hand. Its size, shape, position, and mobility can be estimated.

The examining finger is moved towards one fornix and the hand on the abdomen is moved to the same side. The ovary may be felt (Fig 11); the normal ovary is tender when palpated bimanually. The normal fallopian tube is not palpable. The other lateral fornix is checked and the finger is moved into the posterior fornix to examine the pouch of Douglas. The finger is examined for blood and discharge when it is withdrawn. If a vaginal examination is impossible a rectal one may be done.

Troubleshooting

Vaginismus, a tightening of the levator muscles, can make the use of a speculum impossible – for example, it may not be possible to enter the vagina, or tightening of the muscles after the speculum is in position may cause the patient considerable pain. Do not proceed with the examination if it is painful. Try to understand the reason for the difficulty.

241

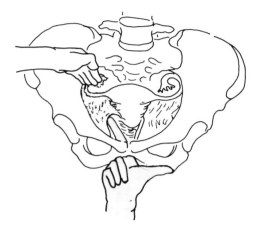

FIG 11   Position of hands during bimanual pelvic examination

The specimen

Smears should be fixed with the fluid available – usually equal parts of absolute alcohol and methylated ether. Transport medium for swabs is supplied by the laboratory and must be stored at the recommended temperature. A culture plate may be used for the investigation of gonorrhoea.

Labelling

The date and time that the specimens were taken must be written on both the form and the specimen. On the form write details about the patient, the identity of the specimen, from where it was collected, the clinical details, and which antibiotics have been given and when.

Aftercare

When the patient is dressed it is advisable to discuss the clinical findings with her and tell her what tests are being done, how long the results will be, and the arrangements for follow up.

Interpretation of results

When the results of a cervical smear test will be available depends on the local cytology service. Usually swab results will be available in a week but some, such as actinomycosis, will take much longer.

24 Proctoscopy and sigmoidoscopy

DJ JONES

Proctoscopy and sigmoidoscopy play a fundamental role in the investigation and management of all patients with anal and large bowel symptoms. Proctoscopy examines the anus and lower rectum; rigid sigmoidoscopy examines the rectum and lower sigmoid colon; flexible sigmoidoscopy examines the colon up to 60 cm from the anal margin.

Equipment

Proctoscopy and rigid sigmoidoscopy can be performed using either disposable plastic or reusable metal instruments. Disposable instruments are more practical in busy clinics, releasing staff from the task of cleaning instruments.

Proctoscopes

These are about 7 cm in length and 2 cm in diameter (Fig 1). The end should be oblique, to allow the walls of the lower rectum and anal canal to be seen clearly. Proctoscopes with an attached fibreoptic light source give better illumination and are more reliable than either proctoscopes with battery powered light sources or those dependent on external illumination.

Rigid sigmoidoscopes

A rigid sigmoidoscope is a straight tube, usually 25 cm in length and about 2 cm in diameter, with a rounded end (Fig 2). A light

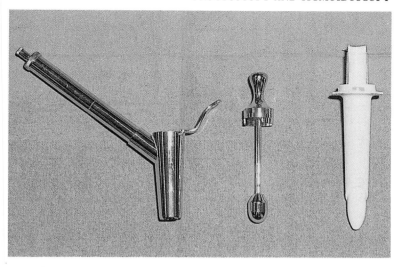

FIG 1 Proctoscopes: disposable plastic proctoscope with the obturator in position (right). Reusable metal proctoscope and obturator; a side blade opposite the handle slides out to facilitate treatment of haemorrhoids (middle and left)

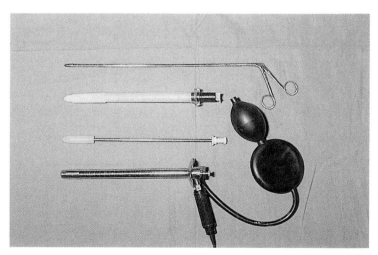

FIG 2 Rigid sigmoidoscopes: biopsy forceps (upper); disposable sigmoidoscope and its obturator (middle); reusable metal sigmoidoscope with attached light source and bellows (lower)

245

source and bellows to inflate the bowel are connected to the eyepiece. The eyepiece is usually detachable and magnifies the view of the mucosa twofold. Biopsy forceps, suction cannulas, long "cotton buds", and other instruments can be introduced by opening a hinged window in the eyepiece. A centimetre scale on the shaft of the instrument allows the distance from the anal margin to any abnormality to be measured. Smaller sigmoidoscopes are available for children and patients with narrow anal canals. Wider sigmoidoscopes are used for operative procedures, such as snaring polyps.

Flexible sigmoidoscopes

These give an excellent view of the large bowel up to 60 cm from the anus. About two thirds of large bowel neoplasms fall within this range. Flexible sigmoidoscopes (Fig 3) are much more expensive than rigid instruments and have to be cleaned and maintained by trained staff. Therefore, the use of fibreoptic instruments tends to be restricted to endoscopy units and/or operating rooms. Video-endoscopes, or video cameras attached to optical endoscopes, allow the endoscopy to be performed using a television monitor rather than by direct vision. This is more comfortable for the endoscopist, more interesting for the attendant staff, useful for

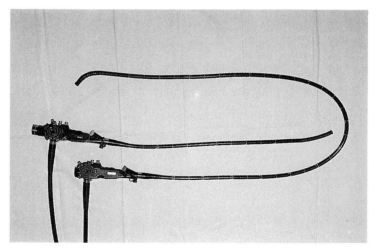

FIG 3   Flexible instruments: colonoscope (outer); flexible sigmoidoscope (inner)

teaching, and avoids the problem of contamination of the face when moving the hand between the scope and the controls. Attached videoprinters allow photographs to be taken to record significant findings.

Bowel preparation

The initial examination should be performed without bowel preparation because this may evoke inflammatory changes and mimic mild proctitis. If the rectum is loaded with faeces a glycerin suppository or phosphate enema can be administered and the examination repeated once the rectum has emptied. Bowel preparation is essential to perform a full flexible sigmoidoscopy and a phosphate enema is usually sufficient. Formal bowel preparation, as for colonoscopy, is sometimes necessary. This involves administering clear fluids and a strong purgative such as sodium picosulphate, on the eve of the examination.

Patient preparation

Patients do not relish undergoing proctoscopy or sigmoidoscopy because of a combination of anxiety and embarrassment. A gentle approach to the patient is essential and fears should be allayed by prior explanation of the procedure. Patients are warned that they may feel they are losing control of their bowels during the examination, but an accident is unlikely. They should also be warned that they will feel a degree of abdominal discomfort and bloating resulting from insufflation of the colon.

Proctoscopy and sigmoidoscopy are usually well tolerated and sedation or general anaesthesia is rarely necessary. If sedation is needed for flexible sigmoidoscopy, a small dose of intravenous midazolam (2·5 mg or 5 mg) or diazepam (Diazemuls) (5 mg) may be administered. The patient should then be monitored using pulse oximetry and oxygen given if the patient's saturation falls. General anaesthesia is indicated for those with painful anal lesions and when an operative procedure is planned.

Position

The patient is placed in the left lateral position, with the hips and knees flexed and the feet lying on the opposite side of the examination couch. The examination is easier if a small cushion or folded blanket is placed under the lower buttocks, which should project a little over the edge of the couch. A protective drape or sheet is tucked under the buttocks to prevent soiling of the couch. Care should be taken at the conclusion of the examination to prevent the patient falling when sitting up. The lithotomy position is often used for patients examined under general anaesthesia.

Technique

The equipment should be ready and checked before starting the procedure. It is useful to wear two gloves on the right hand. The outer glove is discarded after performing a digital examination and introducing the instrument. All examinations commence with a careful inspection of the perineum and anus in a good light. Perineal descent, rectal prolapse, and prolapsing haemorrhoids and tumours may become evident on asking the patient to bear down. If an anal fissure is present, digital and endoscopic examination may be too painful to tolerate without a general anaesthetic.

Common findings on inspection

- Excoriation in pruritus ani
- Anal skin tags
- Anal warts
- Anal fistulae
- Anal fissures
- Perianal abscess
- Prolapsed haemorrhoids
- Rectal prolapse
- Perineal descent
- Anal cancer

A digital examination is performed using a gloved and well lubricated finger. The quantity and consistency of faeces and anal tone at rest and when squeezing are noted. The prostate or cervix is palpated along with any extrarectal lesions. Important palpable abnormalities include rectal polyps and cancers. The withdrawn finger is inspected for blood, mucus, and pus and the nature of the faeces noted.

Proctoscopy

The proctoscope is passed with the obturator in place. The uppermost buttock is lifted with the left hand and the instrument placed on the anal margin and directed towards the umbilicus. The sphincter usually yields spontaneously, allowing the proctoscope to be pushed through with ease.

The obturator is removed and the lower rectum and anal canal inspected. The proctoscope is slowly withdrawn through the anal canal, as it is rotated and angled from side to side, to obtain a complete view of the haemorrhoidal cushions, dentate line, and anal canal. The proctoscope may need to be passed two or three times for complete assessment, the obturator being fitted each time the instrument is introduced. Prolapsing haemorrhoids (Fig 4) and mucosa may be demonstrated by asking the patient to bear down as the proctoscope is withdrawn.

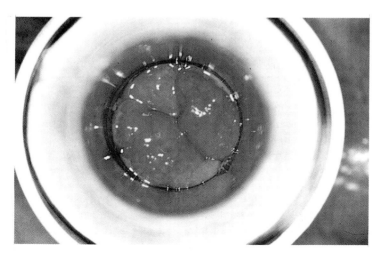

FIG 4   Haemorrhoids seen bulging into the lumen of a proctoscope

> ## Common findings on proctoscopy
>
> Haemorrhoids
> Anal fissures
> Anal fistulae
> Anal polyps
> Anal warts
> Proctitis
> Rectal tumours

Rigid sigmoidoscopy

The examiner stands at the level of the iliac crests and bends to look back towards the anus. The couch should be kept free of dirty swabs and instruments which might come into contact with the head while manipulating and looking down the sigmoidoscope. The instrument is introduced in the same manner as a proctoscope with the obturator held in place with the thumb. Once through the anal canal, the obturator is removed and the eyepiece, light source, and bellows connected.

The instrument is usually held and advanced with the left hand, as the right hand squeezes the bellows. The sigmoidoscope is advanced along the lumen of the rectum, displacing the mucosal folds by gentle angulation of the instrument from side to side during inflation of the bowel. Three or four puffs of the bellows are usually sufficient. The sigmoidoscope should not be pushed forwards if the lumen ahead is not visible.

There is no sequence of specific movements of the rigid sigmoidoscope which guarantee full instrument insertion in all patients. Provided the lumen is visible, the direction for advance is usually obvious and becomes easier with experience. The rectosigmoid junction, which lies about 15 cm from the anal margin, is usually reached; further progress may be easy or difficult depending on the individual patient. Care is needed to negotiate the rectosigmoid junction to minimise discomfort from distortion of the anus and stretching of the colonic wall. Once the sigmoidoscope is manoeuvred beyond this angle, it is usually possible to complete the examination. Pride is not lost if the rectosigmoid cannot be negotiated or the full length of a rigid sigmoidoscope cannot be inserted.

If a more proximal colonic examination is indicated, then a flexible sigmoidoscopy, colonoscopy, or barium enema should be considered.

The best view of the mucosa is obtained while slowly withdrawing the sigmoidoscope, angulating it from side to side. Small polyps, for example, are easily missed when introducing the instrument. Once the examination has been completed, the bowel should be deflated by detaching the eyepiece or opening the window before removal of the sigmoidoscope.

Biopsy samples of protuberant lesions can be taken with impunity, but mucosal biopsies using rigid forceps should only be taken below the peritoneal reflection, which is approximately 10 cm from the anal margin. The biopsy should not be avulsed. Once the bite has been taken, the jaws are held closed as the forceps are rotated through 360°, until the biopsy detaches.

Common findings on sigmoidoscopy

- Polyps
- Carcinomas
- Diverticular openings
- Proctitis
- Colitis

Flexible sigmoidoscopy

A flexible sigmoidoscope has two wheels to steer the tip up and down or from left to right, and two valves to inflate and aspirate the bowel respectively. With practice, it is possible to operate the valves and both wheels with the left hand, using the right hand to advance and withdraw the instrument. The right hand quickly becomes contaminated and is best kept away from the controls and face if using direct vision. Sometimes it is useful to ask an assistant to steady the instrument.

The tip is passed through the anus and the bowel is gently distended with air. The instrument is advanced and steered along the bowel keeping the lumen in view. It is usually easier and less

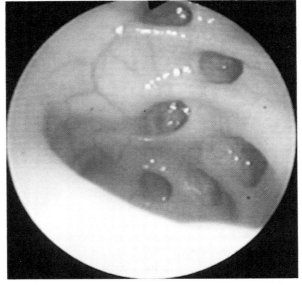

FIG 5   Multiple diverticular openings just proximal to the rectosigmoid junction

painful to negotiate the rectosigmoid junction with a flexible sigmoidoscope than it is with a rigid instrument.

The mucosa may appear normal, inflamed, or ulcerated. Polyps and carcinomas are usually obvious. Blood stained faeces may indicate a lesion in the more proximal colon not reached by sigmoidoscopy. Diverticular pits (Fig 5) may be reached on rigid sigmoidoscopy, but are more commonly seen on flexible sigmoidoscopy. It can be difficult to identify the true lumen in patients with marked diverticulosis, and care is needed to avoid perforating the colon.

25 Ear syringing

S CARNE

Wax (cerumen) is the secretion of the glands in the outer third of the external auditory meatus (Fig 1). Its consistency may be affected by atmospheric pollution. Normally it is expelled by ordinary chewing movements, but in some patients this does not happen. The wax then accumulates and may eventually block the external auditory meatus.

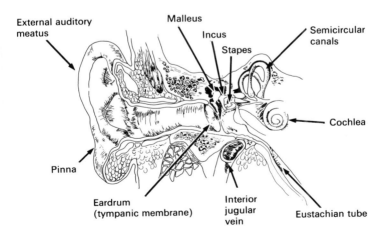

FIG 1   The ear

Indications

Indications

Symptomatic
    Hearing loss: acute and gradual onset
    Earache
    Cough
    Giddiness
Asymptomatic

Symptomatic

1 Hearing loss:
  (a) acute onset: water in the ear may cause sudden swelling of the wax (for example, when swimming under water), which usually brings the patient rapidly to the doctor;
  (b) gradual onset: the hearing loss may go unnoticed by the patient for a long time.
2 Earache: when the wax is pressing on the drum.
3 Cough: when the wax is pressing on the auricular branch of the vagus nerve.
4 Giddiness: sometimes present when there is an obstruction by wax in one meatus only.

Asymptomatic

Wax is frequently seen on routine examination. If the examination is for an insurance or pre-employment medical it may be necessary to remove the wax to ascertain whether (1) the hearing is normal and (2) the drum is perforated. Plugs of wax that do not block the meatus (and hence cannot affect the hearing) and still enable the drum to be seen may safely be left. Sometimes a thin film of wax on the drum (not painful) may give the impression that there is a perforation.

Note: **the ordinary process of syringing when the middle ear is not inflamed often causes a temporary redness of the drum, which may confuse the diagnosis**

Contraindications

The presence of a perforation is a contraindication. Unfortunately, many patients are unaware of the perforation and it may not be identified until after the ear has been syringed. If necessary a prophylactic antibiotic should be administered systematically. Otitis externa is usually regarded as a contraindication because water can aggravate it. Nevertheless, many experienced doctors still syringe the ears when this condition is present but would always be careful gently to mop the meatus dry and might also instil some steroid drops (for example, betamethasone) twice daily for three or four days after syringing.

Wax in the ears of children poses special problems. Syringing the ears in a child is never easy and is particularly difficult when the child is ill; also the procedure is not free from risk of trauma, especially if the child is fractious. Many experienced practitioners prefer to treat the suspected diagnosis rather than risk physical and emotional trauma.

Equipment

Equipment

- Syringe
- Water
- Towels
- Collecting bucket
- Wax hook
- Lighting
- Wax softening agents

Syringe

Most ear syringes are about 18 cm long excluding the nozzle and hold about 120 ml of water. For many years, the author has used a shorter, but stouter, syringe, which is easier to balance in the hand. Regrettably, this type of syringe is not at present available commercially. Some operators have found that a Water Pik, or similar irrigation device (Fig 2), is also useful for syringing ears. Alternatively, a Higginson syringe may serve the purpose provided too

255

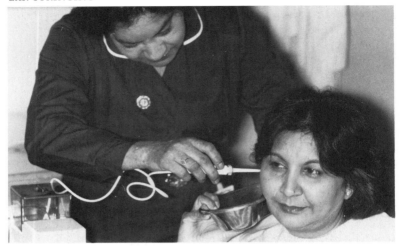

FIG 2 Ear syringing with automatic irrigation device. Note patient holding kidney dish and towel wrapped around the neck and shoulders

great a pressure is not exerted. Whatever instrument is used, sterility is not necessary.

Water

Plain tap water may be used and should be at or slightly above body temperature. The use of sodium bicarbonate in the water is not essential. Water that is too hot or too cold will stimulate the semicircular canals and may cause vertigo, nausea, and vomiting.

Towels

Traditionally a rubber or plastic apron is wrapped round the patient's neck to protect his or her clothes. The cost of laundering cloth towels normally prohibits their use, but paper towels are a satisfactory substitute. They may be tucked inside the collar and will soak up most, if not all, of any water that spills.

Collecting bucket

A Noot's tank is the most convenient, but if one is not available a kidney dish will do. The main disadvantage of the kidney dish is its habit of tipping over when almost full.

Wax hook

A wax hook (Jobson–Horne) is useful to lift out a plug of wax

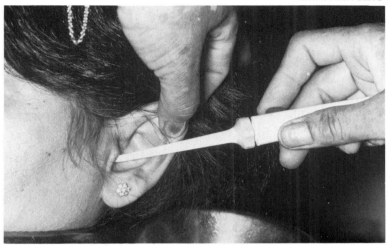

FIG 3   Pinna pulled up and back to straighten the external auditory meatus

that remains obstinately in sight but keeps falling back or one that is stuck to the side wall of the meatus. With many patients, experienced operators can remove all the ear wax with a hook without recourse to syringing.

Lighting

A source of light, either a battery auroscope or a lamp, speculum, and head mirror, is essential for examining the ear before, during, and after the procedure. If a wax hook is to be used in the depths of the external auditory meatus, a head mirror and speculum have an advantage over an electric auroscope in leaving one hand completely free to manipulate the hook.

Wax softening agents

It is usually possible to syringe wax from an ear without any preparation, but first softening the wax eases the process. Sodium bicarbonate eardrops are effective. Alternatively, olive or almond oil or one of the proprietary preparations may be used. After any of these has been used for 2–5 days syringing may sometimes not be necessary. Some of the proprietary preparations, however, may cause otitis externa.

Procedure

If the indications for removing wax are not urgent, prescribe a suitable solvent (for example, sodium bicarbonate ear drops) to be used in the affected ear(s) night and morning for 2–5 days and ask the patient to return at the end of that time. Alternatively, an immediate attempt to remove the wax may be made with a hook or by syringing the ear without preparation. The application of a softening agent for even half an hour before syringing may offer some benefit.

Have the patient sit comfortably in a chair, with the coat removed and a paper towel or plastic apron wrapped round the neck (Fig 2). The patient's cooperation is highly desirable if the meatus and drum are not to be damaged and water is not to be squirted all over the patient, the operator, and the rest of the room. Ask the patient to hold the Noot's tank below the ear, slotting the lobe into the groove. It is easier if the patient holds the tank to the right ear with the left hand and vice versa. This also reduces the risk of the patient knocking the operator's arm away.

When all is ready fill the syringe with water. Be sure no air remains in the syringe, as the sound of bubbles may be frightening to the patient. Pull the pinna up and back to straighten the external meatus (Fig 3). Put the top of the nozzle at the edge of the external auditory meatus, pointed in the direction of the eardrum but slightly backwards and downwards (towards the patient's occiput). Some operators squirt the water in short bursts; others empty each syringeful in one or two actions. The jet of water should pass behind the wax and return into the tank. Sooner or later it will bring with it the lump of wax either intact or in fragments (often several large fragments: hence the need to inspect the ear during the procedure to ensure that all the wax has been cleared).

Water remaining in the meatus will restrict the view and should be gently mopped out with a pledget of cotton wool or paper tissue, but do not damage the eardrum in trying to make sure that the ear is perfectly dry. A small pledget of cotton wool may be left between the tragus and anti-tragus to mop up the last drops, but does not block the meatus.

When the first ear has been freed of wax turn the patient round slowly in the chair (rapid movement can cause giddiness) and proceed in the same way with the other ear.

Complications

The most experienced operators sometimes fail to remove all the wax, even in the most cooperative patient and after using a softening agent. If the wax cannot be removed first time have the patient continue to use the softening agent for at least another seven days before repeating the procedure. If it again fails ask a more experienced operator to try; alternatively, refer the patient to an ENT surgeon. Rarely, a general anaesthetic may be necessary.

If the meatus is scratched it will bleed. This is particularly likely to occur if a wax hook is used by an inexperienced operator. The blood should be gently mopped up with cotton wool. Otitis externa is always a risk, but this may be reduced by careful drying (described above). If an already affected meatus is syringed the local application of steroid drops for one or two days after syringing reduces the risk of any further exacerbation.

Appendix: Aseptic technique and wound dressing

S HUGHES

Definition

An aseptic technique is a method of carrying out sterile procedures so as to minimise the risk of introducing infection. This is achieved by the sterility of the equipment and a no touch method. Scrupulous aseptic technique should always be used for wound care, making surgical incisions, and for all invasive procedures.

Where should aseptic techniques take place?

A designated treatment area is best but for many procedures the bedside is acceptable – avoiding meal times or when ward cleaning is in progress.

Open windows near the patient should be closed, the area needed for the trolley cleared, and bedside screens drawn shut.

The trolley

Trolleys required for aseptic techniques should be used for those purposes only. Usually these trolleys are stored in the clinical room area when not in use. Immediately before setting the trolley with equipment to be used, it should be cleaned thoroughly (Fig 1). Hospital policies can vary slightly and may differ from the method described here. Nurses usually undertake trolley preparation, and perform or assist with the procedure.

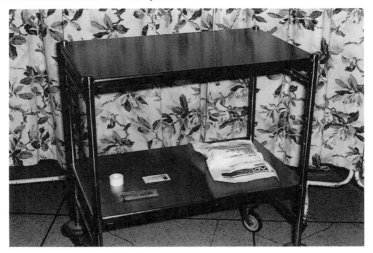

FIG 1   Trolley with dressing pack, Alcowipe, tape, and antiseptic solution on lower shelf

---

Preparation of a trolley

- Wash hands (see Fig 4)
- Apply small amount of liquid detergent to upper surface of trolley and, using a damp paper towel, spread over active surfaces. Pay particular attention to legs and both shelf areas; discard towel
- Rinse with second damp towel; discard towel
- Dry areas fully using a further towel; discard
- The equipment to be used is then obtained, checked, and placed on the lower shelf

---

Example – change of dressing

Equipment

All items should be checked and obtained as below.

Dressing pack

- An outer bag with inner packaging containing four plastic dissecting forceps
- Cotton wool balls × 6

- Gauze × 4 pieces
- 2 gallipots
- 2 dressing towels

The pack should be inspected for damage or tears to the outer covering; ensure that the pack is sealed, sterile, dry, and not outside expiry date.

Alcowipe

An alcohol impregnated towel to cleanse upper shelf. Check packet intact.

Antiseptic solution

Check that you have the correct antiseptic solution, that the container is not damaged, and that its expiry date has not been reached. If an iodine containing solution is to be used, ensure that the patient is not allergic to iodine.

Tape

The adhesive tape to be used should be clean and the material satisfactory for the type of dressing to be secured.

Sellotape should be applied to one of the front trolley legs for attachment of a disposable bag (Fig 2).

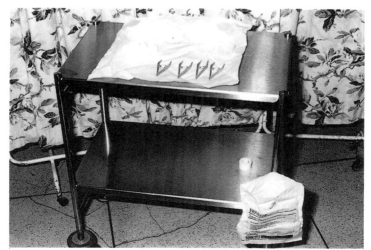

FIG 2   Cleaned trolley with opened dressing pack and disposal bag taped in place

Technique

Equipment

- Trolley
- Dressing pack
- Saline solution
- Adhesive
- Sellotape

Preparation

- Wash hands
- Prepare trolley
- Set lower shelf
- Transport trolley to patient
- Prepare area – assistant can undertake this
- Dresser and assistant to wash hands
- Assistant, standing behind trolley, opens Alcowipe packet and discards outer cover on to lower shelf
- Opening Alcowipe fully place to front edge and side of upper shelf; using palm of hand over the wipe, sweep continuously across surface from right to left working front to back and covering all the area. The Alcowipe is now discarded
- Assistant opens dressing pack at upper end of content bag without touching inside of packet; and holding the outside of the bag the inside parcel is dropped onto upper shelf
- Assistant then attaches bag using sellotape to front of trolley. Inserts Alcowipe/packet into this new disposal bag
- Dresser opens pack using only edges of paper and fully extends all corners
- Dresser takes forceps and arranges pack, gallipots, swabs, gauze, and remaining forceps (Fig 3)
- Assistant opens solutions to be used and pours into gallipots

264

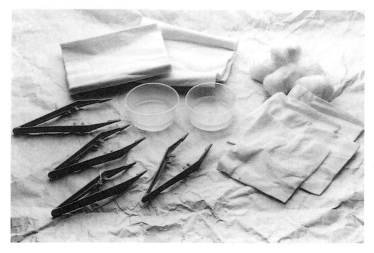

FIG 3   Dressing pack contents arranged in an orderly fashion

Dressing the wound

- Assistant loosens old dressing, lifting all tape from skin, and then washes hands
- Dresser removes dressing with forceps and discards both into bag
- Taking forceps in other hand dresser then picks up a new pair
- Dressing towels are then applied around the wound to form a sterile field
- Assess wound
- Moisten swab with antiseptic solution
- Swab white cotton wool down length of wound once only top to bottom
- Discard swab
- Repeat as necessary
- Dry wound
- Discard forceps used to swab wound
- Apply gauze directly to wound
- Secure with tape

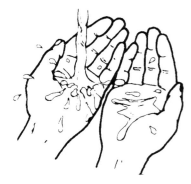

1 Wet hands and forearms thoroughly, apply 5 ml surgical scrub

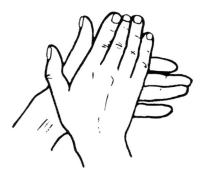

2 Rub palm to palm

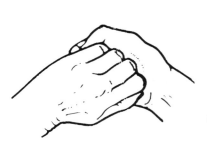

5 Backs of fingers to opposing palms with fingers interlocked

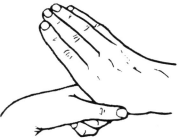

6 Rotational rubbing of right thumb clasped in left palm and vice versa

FIG 4   Hand washing technique

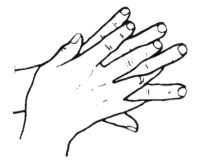

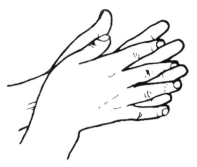

3 Right palm over left dorsum and left palm over right dorsum

4 Palm to palm fingers interlaced

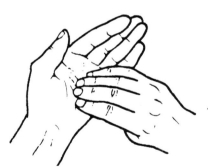

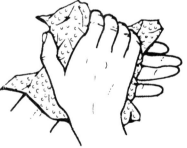

7 Rotational rubbing, backwards and forwards with clasped fingers of right hand in left palm and vice versa

8 Rinse and dry hands and fore-arms thoroughly

Disposal

- Remove towels and discard
- Make patient comfortable
- Wrap pack or remaining contents up and discard into bag. (Gallipots may be resterilised)
- Remove bag and seal
- Dispose of trolley. Dispose of dressing bag into designated receptacle for burning

---

Warning

Make sure all sharps are separately disposed of in a "sharps' container"

Other aseptic procedures

The large majority of practical procedures described in this book are invasive. Aseptic technique is of fundamental importance in ensuring that the patient does not suffer complications from infection introduced by the invasive procedure. The aseptic technique of wound dressing described here embodies the principles that should be adhered to in all invasive procedures.

Index